Diabetic Sweet Treats

Karin Cadwell, Ph.D., R.N.

Foreword by John F. Coughlin, M.D., Ph.D.
Medical Director, Joslin Diabetes Center/Falmouth

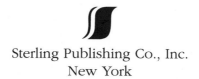

Sterling Publishing Co., Inc.
New York

Acknowledgments

This book would not have been possible without the many taste testers and critics who so unselfishly ate kisses, napoleons, pavlovas, and cream puffs. Thanks to all of you!

Thanks especially to my wonderful husband, Chuck, who is unfailing in his help, and to Hannah Steinmetz, my editor at Sterling.

Library of Congress Cataloging-in-Publication Data

Cadwell, Karin
    Diabetic sweet treats / Karin Cadwell ; foreword by John F. Coughlin.
      p.   cm.
    Includes index.
    ISBN 0-8069-5968-1
    1. Diabetes—Diet therapy—Recipes. 2. Desserts. I. Title.
RC662.C315 1997
641.5'6314–dc21   97-13977
                                            CIP

10 9 8 7 6 5 4 3 2 1

Published by Sterling Publishing Company, Inc.
387 Park Avenue South, New York, N.Y. 10016
© 1997 by Karin Cadwell
Distributed in Canada by Sterling Publishing
C/o Canadian Manda Group, One Atlantic Avenue, Suite 105
Toronto, Ontario, Canada M6K 3E7
Distributed in Great Britain and Europe by Cassell PLC
Wellington House, 125 Strand, London WC2R 0BB, England
Distributed in Australia by Capricorn Link (Australia) Pty Ltd.
P.O. Box 6651, Baulkham Hills, Business Centre, NSW 2153, Australia
Manufactured in the United States of America
All rights reserved

Sterling ISBN 0-8069-5968-1

Contents

FOREWORD 5

INTRODUCTION 7

DRINKS 11

MOSTLY FRUIT 16

ICE CREAM AND FROZEN TREATS 22

PHYLLO DOUGH 28

PUDDING 52

ROLL-UPS 59

MERINGUES 69

ICE BOX PIES 84

GELATIN 100

CREAM PUFFS 110

DRESSED-UP ANGELS 117

BAKED GOODIES 126

EXCHANGE LISTS FOR MEAL PLANNING 143

INDEX 155

Foreword

Unlike short-term crash diets, which have proven to be ineffective in the long run, changes in eating habits are a positive step towards a healthier, happier lifestyle. They make you look and feel better and significantly reduce the risk of a variety of illnesses. Far from being a punishment, they reap innumerable rewards. For example, a recent large nationwide study indicated that when blood sugars were lowered, people with type I diabetes reduced diabetic eye complications by 54 to 76 percent, kidney complications by 39 to 54 percent, and nerve problems by 60 percent.

Many patients who are diabetic or who for other reasons have problems controlling their blood pressure, blood sugar levels, cholesterol, or weight have come to my office looking for solutions to their health problems. Most of them have already tried a variety of "quick fix" schemes and have either given up all hope of living a so-called "normal" life or are still searching for a magic panacea. They fear being put on the dreaded "diet," considering it to be more of a punishment than a cure. They couldn't be more wrong.

Let's not forget that a diet that's good for someone with diabetes is good for someone with a heart condition, a cholesterol problem, or a weight problem. In fact, it's just plain good for anyone!

As Karin Cadwell proves in this remarkable cookbook, choosing a healthier eating plan does not mean you have to sacrifice taste, satisfaction, or fun. Packed with mouthwatering desserts, this volume is a powerful tool to help anyone, diabetic or not, in developing a healthier way of living. The recipes are easy to follow and yield delicious, wholesome results that the whole family will love.

Enjoy!

John F. Coughlin, M.D., Ph.D.
Medical Director
Joslin Diabetes Center/Falmouth

Introduction

Diabetic Sweet Treats is probably different from other cookbooks for diabetics you've read or used because I believe that just about everyone can benefit from low-fat, low-calorie, controlled-carbohydrate desserts. The recipes in this book are meant to be served to your whole family, everyone at the birthday party, or displayed with pride at the potluck supper. I think you will find these desserts delicious enough, attractive enough, and easy enough to make so that you will no longer make two desserts—one for the diabetic and one for everyone else. I make one fabulous dessert everyone can enjoy.

My thinking about diabetic sweet treats began when I was a young girl and my grandfather "got sugar diabetes," as the family said. As a result, my grandmother brought my grandfather's desserts, wrapped in waxed paper, whenever they went out to dinner. My grandmother was a renowned cook and over the years developed many special recipes my grandfather enjoyed, but they weren't shared around. Dinners and special occasions were two-dessert affairs, often plain cake for my grandfather and homemade pastry for the rest of us.

Tom Martin, my parents' good friend, has been on a diabetic diet for as long as I can remember. Over the years there have been countless occasions, from Cub Scout "Blue and Golds" to 50th anniversaries, that feature desserts and sweet treats. At buffets, especially, Tom's wife, Jean, or my mother would peruse the possibilities and tell Tom what he could eat. Often the news was that unless Jean had brought something, Tom was out of luck. Other friends would try to come up with something for Tom when he was going to be a dinner guest. My mother, whose father was on a strict diabetic diet for many years, often got telephone calls asking: "Jean and Tom are coming for dinner this weekend. Do you have any ideas about dessert for Tom?" Often, if the hostess spent her creative talents on the rest of the guests, Tom ended up with "diet" gelatin dessert.

Recently, my mother turned 75. She's been on a diabetic diet for many years, and, when I was planning her big party, a major consideration was that I wanted her to be able to choose from attractive and delicious treats. After all, it was *her* birthday. So, I made only desserts and treats suitable for her fairly strict diet. She was thrilled and so were her guests, all of whom appreciated being treated to luscious low-fat, low-calorie, limited-carbohydrate party food. Many of those recipes are in this book.

Many of the recipes in this book are from scratch. They call for everyday ingredients, many of which you probably already have on hand. They don't usually demand a trip to the supermarket. Other recipes require convenience foods, such as pudding, gelatin mixes, or frozen low-fat non-dairy topping. I have only used ingredients I feel sure are available in every grocery store. I also tried to make your treat-making easier by using appropriate "ready made" foods, such as angel food cakes. Supermarket angel food cakes are very low in fat and (compared to other dessert foods) low in carbohydrates, because they are mostly egg whites and air. Dressing up angel food cakes is a fast and foolproof way to a sweet treat.

Although many of the recipes are quick and easy, some, such as tiramisu, are more complex. Don't be put off by the length of the ingredients list or the directions. Take the recipes step-by-step and you'll be thrilled with the results. This book has a whole chapter on meringues, featuring the classic Pavlova. This is an ideal dessert, tempting and beautiful yet easy and healthful. Even if you have never seen a Pavlova before, try it. You'll be delighted. Just be sure to read the introductory recipe or section at the beginning of each chapter to orient you and point out any special considerations.

This book is organized by the central technique or ingredient featured in each chapter. Phyllo dough, for example, is a great ingredient for diabetic sweet treats, but *please* follow my low-fat, low-calorie instructions, not the melted-butter ones on the phyllo box!

So that beginner cooks will be able to prepare these wonderful treats, I have tried not to use specialized equipment. However, for some recipes you need a blender or food processor, because chopping and mixing by hand just doesn't produce the same results as by machine. In a few cases, I used an ice cream maker.

I've tried to give you a choice about which sugar substitute to use. In many cases, any of the three available basic substitutes will work: aspartame (Nutrasweet, Equal); saccharin (Sweet n' Low, Sugar Twin); acesulfame-K or Ace-K (Sweet-One). Some people prefer one taste over another and when it doesn't matter, I just call for sugar substitute. Other times, especially when heat or freezing is involved, I indicate the one that works best when I prepare the recipe. These chemicals can change flavor and become bitter with different temperatures. Here is a chart that will help you make substitutions.

Guide to Approximate Equivalents
Amount of Artificial Sweeteners to substitute for sugar

Sugar	Acesulfame-K	Aspartame	Saccharin
2 t	1 pkt.	1 pkt. or ¼ t	1 pkt. or ⅕ t
1 T	1¼ pkt.	1½ pkt. or ½ t	1⅓ pkt. or ⅓ t
¼ cup	3 pkts.	6 pkts. or 1¾ t	3 pkts. or 1⅙ t
⅓ cup	4 pkts.	8 pkts. or 2½ t	4 pkts. or 1¼ t
½ cup	6 pkts.	12 pkts. or 3½ t	6 pkts. or 2 t
⅔ cup	8 pkts.	16 pkts. or 5 t	8 pkts. or 2½ t
¾ cup	9 pkts.	18 pkts. or 5¼ t	9 pkts. or 3½ t
1 cup	12 pkts.	24 pkts. or 7¼ t	12 pkts. or 4 t

Please keep in mind that aspartame (marketed as Equal or NutraSweet) must be added after cooking. I like to store our aspartame with a vanilla bean in little covered containers. I do this with Equal Measure (a concentrated form of aspartame) and NutraSweet Spoonful (the measures-like-sugar-type of aspartame).

If your supermarket doesn't carry Acesulfame-K, which is marketed as Sweet One, you can call 1–800–544–8610, or write to Stadt Corporation, 60 Flushing Avenue, Brooklyn, NY 11205, for information about how to get it.

One of the reasons I use different sugar substitutes is that my taste testers tend to find that heat-treated foods containing aspartame taste bitter. In most recipes you can substitute one brand of sugar substitute for another according to your individual preference.

Outside the U.S., the same artificial sweeteners tend to be available and are frequently marketed with the same brand names mentioned above. A choice may be a mix of sweeteners marketed in a blend and may include cyclamate. In all cases, these products are reasonably the same equivalents as those listed here. Just be sure to choose a concentrated variety where about one-fifth to one-quarter of a teaspoon is equivalent to two teaspoons of sugar. If the product is sold in a jar, use a quarter of a teaspoon to equal a packet.

I hope you enjoy making and serving these sweet treats. I know you'll be proud to serve them.

Drinks

Vanilla Shake

As good as the ones in your favorite fast-food restaurant.

½ C	skim milk	125 mL
1 C	frozen fat-free non-dairy whipped topping	250 mL
1 T	vanilla extract	15 mL
½ C	crushed ice	125 mL

Place all the ingredients in a blender or food processor. Process at the highest speed until liquefied. Serve immediately.

Yield: 1 serving
Each serving contains:
Calories (Kcal): 165   Total fat (g): 0
Carbohydrates (g): 26   Protein (g) 4
Sodium (mg): 67   Cholesterol (mg): 2
Diabetic exchange: 1½ starch/bread

Pineapple-Mint Drink

If you don't have a fresh pineapple, use canned pineapple packed in its own juice. Drain it first.

½ C	water (or drained pineapple juice)	125 mL
1 C	pineapple, cut into pieces	250 mL
3 whole	oranges, seeded and chopped	3 whole
1 C	crushed ice	250 mL
½ t	mint extract	3 mL

Put all the ingredients into a blender or food processor. Blend at the highest speed until the ice is liquefied.

Yield: 6 servings
Each serving contains:
Calories (Kcal): 44   Total fat (g): .2
Carbohydrates (g): 11   Protein (g): .7
Sodium (mg): 2   Cholesterol (mg): 0
Diabetic exchange: ¾ fruit

Chocolate Frappé

A wonderful chocolaty taste. My daughter Anna loves this drink.

1 env.	hot chocolate mix, no sugar added	1 env.
3 T	hot water	45 mL
1 C	skim milk	250 mL
1 C	crushed ice	250 mL

In a small bowl, combine the hot chocolate mix and water until a smooth paste forms. Put the milk and crushed ice into a food processor or blender. Using a rubber scraper, pour the chocolate paste over the milk and ice mixture. Process at the highest speed until the ice is liquefied. Serve in tall glasses.

Yield: 2 servings
Each serving contains:

Calories (Kcal): 73	Total fat (g): 0.7
Carbohydrates (g): 11	Protein (g): 5
Sodium (mg): 147	Cholesterol (mg): 2
Diabetic exchange: 1 milk	

Butter-Almond Frappé

Do you like butter-almond ice cream? This is a wonderful substitute!

1 C	frozen fat-free non-dairy whipped topping	250 mL
½ t	butter extract	3 mL
½ t	almond extract	3 mL
1 C	crushed ice	250 mL

Put all the ingredients into a food processor or blender. Blend at the highest speed until the ice is liquefied.

Yield: 1 serving
Each serving contains:

Calories (Kcal): 125	Total fat (g): 0
Carbohydrates (g): 20	Protein (g): 0
Sodium (mg): 7	Cholesterol (mg): 0
Diabetic exchange: 1 fruit	

Virgin Piña Colada

This is thick and frothy; imagine yourself sitting beside a pool in the tropics sipping it.

1 C	frozen fat-free non-dairy whipped topping	250 mL
2 T	crushed pineapple in juice, drained	30 mL
1 t	rum extract	5 mL
1 t	coconut extract	5 mL
1 C	crushed ice	250 mL

Place all the ingredients in a food processor or blender. Process at the highest speed until the ice is liquefied.

Yield: 1 serving
Each serving contains:
Calories (Kcal): 40　　　Total fat (g): 0
Carbohydrates (g): 30　　Protein (g): 0.1
Sodium (mg): 7　　　　　Cholesterol (mg): 0
Diabetic exchange: 1½ fruit

Icy Eggnog

Terrific for holiday get-togethers. Serve in punch cups sprinkled with nutmeg or cinnamon.

3 C	skim milk	750 mL
¾ C	egg substitute, liquid	185 mL
1 T	sugar	15 mL
2 pkgs.	sugar substitute	2 pkgs.
1 t	vanilla extract	5 mL
1 C	crushed ice	250 mL

Put all the ingredients in a blender or food processor and process at the highest speed until the ice is liquefied.

Yield: 8 servings
Each serving contains:
Calories (Kcal): 60　　　Total fat (g): 1
Carbohydrates (g): 6　　　Protein (g): 6
Sodium (mg): 91　　　　Cholesterol (mg): 2
Diabetic exchange: ½ milk

Orange Banana Smoothie

As good as it can be. Use sweet oranges and remove the white skin.

2	oranges, peeled and cut into chunks	2
1	ripe banana, peeled and sliced	1
½ C	skim milk	125 mL
1 pkg.	aspartame sweetener	1 pkg.
¼ t	almond extract	2 mL
3	ice cubes	3

Put all the ingredients into a blender or food processor. Blend at the highest speed until smooth. Pour into four glasses. Serve cold.

> Yield: 4 servings
> Each serving contains:
> Calories (Kcal): 69 — Total fat (g): 0.3
> Carbohydrates (g): 16 — Protein (g): 2
> Sodium (mg): 17 — Cholesterol (mg): 1
> Diabetic exchange: 1 starch/bread

Strawberry Smoothie

I've used frozen berries in this with excellent results.

1 C	skim milk	250 mL
¾ C	fresh or sugar-free whole frozen strawberries	185 mL
1 pkg.	sugar substitute	1 pkg.
½ t	lemon extract	3 mL
1 C	crushed ice	250 mL

Put all the ingredients in a blender or food processor. Blend at the highest speed until the ice is liquefied.

> Yield: 4 servings
> Each serving contains:
> Calories (Kcal): 31 — Total fat (g): 0.2
> Carbohydrates (g): 5 — Protein (g): 2
> Sodium (mg): 35 — Cholesterol (mg): 1
> Diabetic exchange: 1 vegetable

Raspberry Frappé

Raspberry extract makes all the difference. Buy it at a specialty food shop since supermarkets carry only the most ordinary flavors.

1 C	raspberry sugar-free soda	250 mL
⅓ C	plain yogurt	80 mL
1 pkg.	sugar substitute	1 pkg.
1 t	raspberry extract	5 mL
½ T	vanilla extract	7.5 mL

Put all the ingredients into a blender or food processor. Blend or process at the highest speed until the ice is liquefied.

Yield: 1 serving
Each serving contains:
Calories (Kcal): 63 — Total fat (g): 2
Carbohydrates (g): 5 — Protein (g): 3
Sodium (mg): 39 — Cholesterol (mg): 10
Diabetic exchange: 1 vegetable; ½ fat

Mocha Frappé

As self-indulgent as those high-fat fancy coffee drinks.

1 env.	sugar-free hot chocolate mix	1 env.
3 T	hot coffee	45 mL
1 C	skim milk	250 mL
1 C	crushed ice	250 mL

Put all the ingredients into a food processor or blender. Process at the highest speed until the ice is liquefied.

Yield: 1 serving
Each serving contains:
Calories (Kcal): 86 — Total fat (g): 0.4
Carbohydrates (g): 12 — Protein (g): 8
Sodium (mg): 134 — Cholesterol (mg): 4
Diabetic exchange: 1 milk

Mostly Fruit

Peach Clafouti

Clafouti is like a cobbler. It's just one dish, easy with fruit and pastry.

1 lb	peaches, sliced	450 g
1 C	skim milk	250 mL
2 whole	egg or equivalent egg substitute	2 whole
2 T	peach-flavored brandy (optional)	30 mL
2 T	sugar	30 mL
2 pkgs.	acesulfame-K	2 pkgs.
½ C	flour	125 mL
¼ t	nutmeg	2 mL

Coat a one-quart (1 L) shallow baking dish with non-stick vegetable cooking spray. Arrange peach slices evenly on the bottom of it.

Put the milk, eggs, brandy (if you are using it), sugar, and acesulfame-K in a blender or food processor. Use a tablespoon (15 mL) measure and remove 1 tablespoon (15 mL) flour from the half-cup (125 mL) measure and mix in the nutmeg. Set aside. Add the ½ cup minus 1 T (125 mL minus 15 mL) flour to the mixture in the blender or food processor and process until smooth. Pour over the peaches.

Sprinkle with the flour-nutmeg mixture. Bake in a preheated 350°F (180°C) oven for 30–35 minutes. The topping will be golden and puffed.

Yield: 6 servings
Each serving contains:

Calories (Kcal): 126	Total fat (g): 2
Carbohydrates (g): 23	Protein (g): 5
Sodium (mg): 248	Cholesterol (mg): 72

Diabetic exchange: 1½ starch/bread

Peach Crème Fraîche

My cousin Ingrid loves this one. She couldn't believe it was so low in calories.

20 oz	peach slices in juice	550 g
1 C	frozen low-fat non-dairy whipped topping	250 mL
1 t	almond extract	5 mL

1 env.	plain gelatin	1 env.	
3 T	water	45 mL	

Drain the peaches. Reserve four slices for garnish. Discard the juice or reserve it for another use. Put the peaches, whipped topping, and almond extract in a blender or food processor. Blend until smooth. In a small saucepan, mix together the gelatin and water. Let stand five minutes. Heat over low flame, stirring constantly until the gelatin is dissolved. Add to the peach mixture. Blend another few seconds. Spoon into four dessert dishes. Refrigerate until serving time. Garnish with the reserved peach slices and additional whipped topping, if desired.

Yield: 4 servings
Each serving contains:
Calories (Kcal): 114　　Total fat (g): 2
Carbohydrates (g): 22　　Protein (g): 2
Sodium (mg): 11　　Cholesterol (mg): 0
Diabetic exchange: 1 starch/bread; ½ fruit

Yogurt Orange Whip

I make this before starting the rest of dinner. By the time we're ready for dessert, it's chilled.

4	oranges, peeled	4	
3 pkgs.	sugar substitute	3 pkgs.	
2 C	lemon or vanilla nonfat yogurt	500 mL	
2 T	walnuts(optional)	30 mL	

Chop the oranges coarsely. Place them in a blender or food processor. Add the sugar substitute and yogurt and process at a high speed until ingredients are well combined. Pour into four dessert dishes. Chill for an hour or two. Just before serving, sprinkle the tops with walnuts if desired.

Yield: 4 servings
Each serving contains:
Calories (Kcal): 65　　Total fat (g): 0.2
Carbohydrates (g): 16　　Protein (g): 1
Sodium (mg): 3　　Cholesterol (mg): 0
Diabetic exchange: 1 fruit

Bananas and Yogurt

The yogurt is like sweetened whipped cream.

4	ripe bananas, peeled	4
3 pkgs.	sugar substitute	3 pkgs.
1 C	nonfat vanilla yogurt	250 mL
2 T	walnuts, chopped (optional)	30 mL

Slice the bananas in half lengthwise. Cut into chunks and place one banana in each serving dish. In a mixing bowl, combine the sugar substitute, yogurt, and vanilla. Put one quarter of the yogurt mixture over the bananas in each dish.

Chill for one hour before serving. Sprinkle with nuts, if desired.

Yield: 4 servings
Each serving contains:

Calories (Kcal): 159	Total fat (g): 0.6
Carbohydrates (g): 37	Protein (g): 4
Sodium (mg): 43	Cholesterol (mg): 1

Diabetic exchange: 1 starch/bread; 1½ fruit

Individual Banana Soufflés

Serve these right away!

6 medium	bananas, ripe and peeled	6 medium
1 T	cornstarch	15 mL
½ C	skim milk	125 mL
1 t	almond extract or	5 mL
1 T	almond liqueur	15 mL
2	egg yolks	2
3	egg whites	3
½ t	confectioners' sugar	3 mL

Puree the bananas. Measure 2 cups (500 mL) for use in this recipe. Combine the cornstarch and skim milk and cook in a heavy-bottomed medium saucepan. Stir constantly until the mixture thickens. Continue stirring and add the extract or liqueur, banana puree, and egg yolks. Bring to a boil. Transfer to a mixing bowl. Cool. Beat the egg whites until stiff but not dry. Fold them into the banana mixture carefully. Spoon the mixture into individual soufflé dishes that have been coated with non-stick vegetable cooking spray. Place them in a preheated 350°F (180°C) oven for

10–15 minutes. Try not to open the oven door during this time. The tops should be brown and the soufflés puffed. Sprinkle the tops with confectioners' sugar.

> Yield: 6 servings
>> Each serving contains:
>> Calories (Kcal): 147 Total fat (g): 2
>> Carbohydrate(g): 29 Protein (g): 5
>> Sodium (mg): 10 Cholesterol (mg): 71
>> Diabetic exchange: 2 starch/bread

Frozen Bananas

Keep these in a plastic bag in the freezer for instant snacks.

2 medium	firm bananas	2 medium
⅓ C	sugar-free chocolate candy, broken up	80 mL
2 T	creamy peanut butter	30 mL
2 T	nuts, chopped and toasted	30 mL

Cut the bananas into four pieces each. Put the pieces on a pan in the freezer for 30 minutes. Melt the chocolate over a very low flame in a small saucepan. Add the peanut butter and stir. Put the chocolate mixture on one plate and the nuts on another. Roll the banana pieces in the chocolate and then the nuts. Return to the freezer to harden the chocolate. Store the pieces in the freezer in a plastic bag.

> Yield: 8 servings
>> Each serving contains:
>> Calories (Kcal): 101 Total fat (g): 5
>> Carbohydrates (g): 14 Protein (g): 2
>> Sodium (mg): 20 Cholesterol (mg): 1
>> Diabetic exchange: 1 starch/bread; 1 fat

Fried Spiced Apples

This is a wonderfully satisfying dessert for a winter evening.

4 large	cooking apples, peeled and cored	4 large
1 t	sugar	5 mL
¼ t	ginger	2 mL
¼ t	cinnamon	2 mL
2 T	butter or margarine	30 mL
1 C	frozen low-fat non-dairy whipped topping	250 mL

Cut the apples into ¼-inch (6 mm) thick slices. On a dinner plate, mix together the sugar, ginger, and cinnamon. In a large, heavy-bottomed frying pan, melt the butter or margarine. Dip the apple slices in the sugar and cinnamon mixture. Fry 3–5 minutes on each side or until lightly browned. Remove slices to a serving dish. Serve immediately with whipped topping.

Yield: 4 servings
Each serving contains:

Calories (Kcal): 176	Total fat (g): 8
Carbohydrates (g): 26	Protein (g): 0.3
Sodium (mg): 58	Cholesterol (mg): 15

Diabetic exchange: 2 fruit; 1½ fat

Marinated Blueberries

Delicious when blueberries are fresh and plentiful.

2 C	fresh blueberries	500 mL
1 t	grated orange rind	5 mL
2 T	Triple Sec or other orange-flavored liqueur	30 mL
2 t	sugar	10 mL
½ C	frozen low-fat non-dairy whipped topping	125 mL

In a shallow mixing bowl, combine the blueberries, orange rind, Triple Sec, and sugar. Toss to coat the berries. Cover loosely and refrigerate for an hour or more. Before serving, mix a few times. Serve with whipped topping.

Yield: 4 servings
Each serving contains:

Calories (Kcal): 69	Total fat (g): 1
Carbohydrates (g): 14	Protein (g): 1
Sodium (mg): 4	Cholesterol (mg): 0

Diabetic exchange: 1 starch/bread

Oranges and Grapes

Make a glamorous-looking fresh dessert with fresh winter fruits.

4	oranges, peeled	4
1 C	grapes, halved and seeded, if necessary	250 mL
¼ C	water	60 mL
1 t	rum flavoring	5 mL
2 pkgs.	sugar substitute	2 pkgs.

Slice the oranges into layers. Arrange with grape halves in a glass serving dish. Mix together the water, flavoring, and sugar substitute.

Pour the mixture over the fruit. Cover the bowl and refrigerate for at least an hour before serving.

Yield: 4 servings
Each serving contains:
Calories (Kcal): 90   Total fat (g): 0.3
Carbohydrates (g): 23   Protein (g): 2
Sodium (mg): 3   Cholesterol (mg): 0
Diabetic exchange: 1 starch/bread; ½ fruit

Piña Colada Sherbet

You don't make this sherbet and freeze it; you freeze the pineapple ahead of time.

20 oz	pineapple chunks in juice, no sugar added	550 g
2 t	coconut extract	10 mL
1 C	frozen low-fat non-dairy whipped topping	250 mL

Drain and freeze the pineapple chunks. Put them into a food processor. If the pineapple sticks to the container, run water on the outside. Add the coconut extract and blend until mushy. Transfer to a medium mixing bowl. Fold in the whipped topping. Serve immediately.

Yield: 4 servings
Each serving contains:
Calories (Kcal): 127   Total fat (g): 2
Carbohydrates (g): 26   Protein (g): 0.6
Sodium (mg): 1   Cholesterol (mg): 0
Diabetic exchange: 2 fruit; ½ fat

Ice Cream and Frozen Treats

Frozen Watermelon Pops

I love this recipe. Even though loads of people are at my house for summer weekends, some watermelon is always left over. I prepare these early in the morning with leftover melon. When the crowd comes back from the beach these pops are ready. To serve on Popsicle sticks, insert sticks after the pops have been in the freezer half an hour or so.

3 C	pureed watermelon	750 mL
1 T	lemon juice	15 mL
1 env.	unflavored gelatin	1 env.
1 pkg.	strawberry gelatin powder, sugar-free	1 pkg.
2 C	frozen low-fat non-dairy whipped topping, softened	500 mL

In a saucepan, combine the watermelon puree, lemon juice, and unflavored gelatin. Set aside for five minutes. Heat over a low flame, stirring until the gelatin dissolves. Remove from the heat and stir in the strawberry gelatin. Mix until smooth and the gelatin is dissolved. Refrigerate for 15 minutes, to bring to room temperature. In a large mixing bowl, fold together the gelatin mixture and whipped topping. Distribute into eight 4-oz (100 g) paper cups. Freeze. To serve, peel back the paper.

Yield: 8 servings
Each serving contains:

Calories (Kcal): 66	Total fat (g): 2
Carbohydrates (g): 9	Protein (g): 1
Sodium (mg): 11	Cholesterol (mg): 0
Diabetic exchange: ½ fruit; ½ fat	

Tropical Banana Pops

These are easy to make. Keep some in the freezer for hot summer afternoons.

4	small bananas, crushed	4
1 t	lemon juice	5 mL
1¼ C	tropical sugar-free drink, from powder	310 mL
1 t	coconut extract or flavoring	5 mL

Put the crushed bananas into a medium bowl. Sprinkle with lemon juice and toss. Mix in the other ingredients. Spoon into six 4-oz (100 g) paper cups. Freeze until firm. To serve, peel back the paper.

Yield: 6 servings
Each serving contains:

Calories (Kcal): 72	Total fat (g): 0.4
Carbohydrates (g): 18	Protein (g): 0.8
Sodium (mg): 1	Cholesterol (mg): 0
Diabetic exchange: 1 fruit	

Tortoni

Low-calorie, low-fat version of the traditional Italian dessert.

⅔ C	ice water	165 mL
⅔ C	dry skim milk	165 mL
¼ C	lemon juice	60 mL
3 pkgs.	sugar substitute	3 pkgs.
2 T	sherry	30 mL
½ t	vanilla extract	3 mL
½ t	almond extract	3 mL
¼ C	sliced toasted almonds (optional)	60 mL
6	maraschino cherries, chopped	6

In an electric mixer bowl or food processor, beat the ice water and dry milk until the mixture begins to be thickened. Add the lemon juice and sugar substitute and beat until thick. Beat in the sherry and extracts. Fold in the toasted almonds, if you are using them, and the cherry pieces. Freeze.

Yield: 4 servings
Each serving contains:

Calories (Kcal): 98	Total fat (g): 0.2
Carbohydrates (g): 15	Protein (g): 7
Sodium (mg): 116	Cholesterol (mg): 4
Diabetic exchange: 1 milk	

Lemon Ice Cream

You don't need an ice cream machine for this one!

1 C	skim milk	250 mL
1 pkg.	lemon gelatin powder, sugar-free	1 pkg.
1 T	lemon juice	15 mL
2 pkgs.	sugar substitute	2 pkgs.
1 C	frozen low-fat non-dairy whipped topping	250 mL
1 t	vanilla extract	5 mL

Scald the milk in a medium saucepan. Stir in the lemon gelatin and the lemon juice. Mix to dissolve the powder. Put the saucepan in the refrigerator to cool but not to set, 15–20 minutes. Stir in the sugar substitute and lemon juice. Fold in the whipped topping and vanilla extract. Blend thoroughly. Freeze in an ice tray until set. Turn the frozen mixture into a food processor or electric mixer bowl. Process until light and fluffy. Return to the freezer tray. Freeze for an additional 3 hours.

> Yield: 4 servings
> Each serving contains:
> Calories (Kcal): 68   Total fat (g): 2
> Carbohydrates (g): 8   Protein (g): 2
> Sodium (mg): 88   Cholesterol (mg): 1
> Diabetic exchange: ½ fruit; ¼ high fat meat

Honeydew Sherbet

If you don't have an ice cream machine, this won't be as creamy, but it will still taste fabulous.

½	medium honeydew melon	½
1¾ C	frozen low-fat non-dairy whipped topping, thawed	435 mL
1 T	Triple Sec (optional)	15 mL
1 dash	aspartame sweetener to taste (optional)	1 dash

Cut the melon in half and remove the seeds. Peel the melon. Scoop the soft pulp into chunks. Puree in a food processor. Measure 1¾ cups (435 mL) of melon puree. Discard any extra, or reserve it for another use. Put the melon into a mixing bowl. Add the whipped topping. Mix to blend. Add the Triple

Sec or aspartame, if desired. Process in an ice cream machine according to the manufacturer's directions.

Yield: 8 servings
Each serving contains:

Calories (Kcal): 63	Total fat (g): 2
Carbohydrates (g): 11	Protein (g): 0.4
Sodium (mg): 8	Cholesterol (mg): 0

Diabetic exchange: ⅔ fruit; ½ fat

Orange Frost

I make this in the summer and freeze it in paper cups for barbecue desserts. This recipe works best with the freezer turned to its coldest setting.

1 C	orange juice	250 mL
2 T	lemon juice	30 mL
1 t	orange flavoring	5 mL
1 C	frozen low-fat non-dairy whipped topping, softened	250 mL

Combine the orange juice and lemon juice in a mixing bowl. Stir in the orange flavoring. Pour the mixture into four freezer-safe dessert dishes (*i.e.,* paper, Pyrex, metal). Freeze. Serve with whipped topping.

Yield: 4 servings
Each serving contains:

Calories (Kcal): 70	Total fat (g): 2
Carbohydrates (g): 11	Protein (g): 1
Sodium (mg): 1	Cholesterol (mg): 0

Diabetic exchange: ⅔ fruit; ½ fat

Mixed Fruit Sherbet

This is really different. If you like fruity desserts you'll love this one.

2 C	strawberries, fresh or whole frozen, thawed	500 mL
1	ripe banana	1
½ C	orange	125 mL
6 pkts.	aspartame sweetener	90 mL
2 C	frozen low-fat non-dairy whipped topping, thawed	500 mL
1½ C	skim milk	375 mL

Wash, hull, and slice the strawberries. Put them in a mixing bowl. Peel and slice the banana. Mash the two fruits together with a fork. Stir in the remaining ingredients and mix until everything is evenly combined. Process in an ice cream machine according to manufacturer's directions.

Yield: 8 servings
Each serving contains:

Calories (Kcal): 92	Total fat (g): 2
Carbohydrates (g): 15	Protein (g): 2
Sodium (mg): 24	Cholesterol (mg): 1
Diabetic exchange: 1 starch/bread	

Strawberry-Banana Frozen Yogurt

If you use an ice cream machine, this will be smoother than if you just freeze it, but it's great either way.

1 pkg. (4 servings)	strawberry-banana sugar-free gelatin mix	1 pkg. (4 servings)
1 C	boiling water	250 mL
½ C	cold water	125 mL
1 C	fresh or frozen strawberries, diced and mashed	250 mL
1 C	low-fat vanilla yogurt	250 mL
2 C	frozen low-fat non-dairy whipped topping, thawed	500 mL

Put the gelatin into a mixing bowl. Add the boiling water. Stir to dissolve. Add the cold water and the strawberries. In another bowl, use a wire whisk to combine the yogurt and whipped topping. Pour the gelatin mixture into the yogurt mixture. Mix thoroughly. Process in an ice cream machine according to manufacturer's directions or pour into a brownie pan and freeze.

Yield: 6 servings
Each serving contains:

Calories (Kcal): 129	Total fat (g): 3
Carbohydrates (g): 10	Protein (g): 14
Sodium (mg): 59	Cholesterol (mg): 1

Diabetic exchange: 1 milk; 1 lean meat

Frozen Strawberry Mousse

Lovely! You'll be proud to serve this.

2 C	fresh strawberries, hulled	500 mL
1 T	sugar	15 mL
½ T	gelatin	7.5 mL
3 T	cold water	45 mL
5 pkgs.	aspartame sweetener	5 pkgs.
2 C	frozen low-fat non-dairy whipped topping	500 mL

Cut the strawberries into a medium bowl. Sprinkle with sugar and set aside. Sprinkle the gelatin over the cold water in the top of a double boiler. Bring the water to a boil in the bottom of the double boiler. Put on the top part of the double boiler and heat the gelatin mixture until it dissolves. Remove from heat. Mash the strawberries. Fold in the gelatin and the whipped topping. Freeze.

Yield: 8 servings
Each serving contains:

Calories (Kcal): 60	Total fat (g): 2
Carbohydrates (g): 9	Protein (g) 0.3
Sodium (mg): 1	Cholesterol (mg): 0

Diabetic exchange: ½ fruit; ½ fat

Phyllo Dough

Phyllo dough is a paper-thin pastry made in the Mediterranean since ancient times. In most recipes phyllo dough is layered and baked to a golden-brown color. Because it has virtually no fat, phyllo is an ideal dough for diabetic desserts and sweet treats.

General Instructions

•Buy phyllo or "Fillo" dough in the freezer section of the supermarket. The dough comes in large rectangular sheets.

•Store the box in the freezer until the day before you want to use it.

•Transfer the unopened box to the refrigerator to thaw overnight.

•Choose a large work surface, such as a kitchen table.

•Wet a dish towel and wring it out thoroughly. You will also need a piece of plastic. I usually use an unused plastic trash bag.

•Open the phyllo dough box and carefully unroll the dough onto your work surface.

•Cover the dough immediately with the plastic and spread the damp towel over on top. This is the key to working with phyllo dough. Don't let it dry out! Don't leave the pile uncovered except when you are removing one sheet from it.

•Roll any unused sheets of phyllo in the plastic it was originally packaged in and refreeze. I usually add an extra plastic layer of wrapping to be sure the sheets don't dry out in the freezer.

•Work phyllo dough one layer at a time. Uncover the pile, remove one sheet, and cover the pile again.

•Use butter-flavored vegetable cooking spray instead of melted butter. This will really help cut down on calories. Start by spraying around the edges. This will help to avoid cracking. Work toward the center. Spray the sheet evenly. You generally put four sheets on top of one another. Don't forget to spray the last sheet. Cut through all four sheets to form 16 rectangular piles each four sheets high. Place these stacks on ungreased cookie sheets (or whatever the recipe calls for) and bake them in a preheated oven. Remove phyllo promptly from the oven. Cool completely.

In the following recipes you'll often use three of these rectangular stacks together with fillings between the stacks to form each napoleon.

I've included some of my favorite phyllo recipes. I think you'll find them easy and delicious.

Hawaiian Napoleon

Zoë and Tim were the major testers for the napoleons. They became engaged in the process. Was it the napoleons?

3 piles	phyllo dough napoleon rectangles (4 deep)	3 piles
¼ C	sugar-free vanilla pudding made with skim milk	60 mL
1 T	pineapple, crushed, in juice	15 mL
1 t	coconut flakes	25 mL
1 t	Strawberry-Kiwi Glaze (p. 30)	25 mL

Bake sheets of phyllo according to the general instructions at the beginning of this chapter. Cut the pile of four sprayed sheets into 16 rectangles. Bake in a preheated 375°F (190°C) oven for 8 minutes. Three of these rectangular piles are used to make each napoleon.

Place one cooked and cooled four-layer rectangular stack on a dessert plate. Spread on the vanilla pudding. Place a second rectangular pile on top of the vanilla pudding. Top this layer with the crushed pineapple. Sprinkle on the coconut. Add the last layer of phyllo. Smooth on the Strawberry-Kiwi Glaze.

> Yield: 1 Hawaiian Napoleon
> Calories (Kcal): 105   Total fat (g): 1
> Carbohydrates (g): 21   Protein (g): 1
> Sodium (mg): 248   Cholesterol (mg): 0
> Diabetic exchange: 1 fruit; ⅓ starch/bread

Strawberry Kiwi Glaze

Glaze Hawaiian Napoleons with this.

¼ C	lemon juice	60 mL
¼ C	water	60 mL
1 T	cornstarch	15 mL
2 t	strawberry-kiwi Crystal Light mix	10 mL

In a small saucepan, mix together the lemon juice, water, and cornstarch. Stir until smooth. Heat over medium heat until the mixture begins to boil. Stirring constantly, lower heat and cook until mixture turns from milky to opaque and thickens. Set aside to cool. Stir in strawberry-kiwi mix. Blend well. Add a few drops of water if the mixture becomes too thick to spread evenly.

> Yield: ½ cup of glaze—25 servings (1 t [5 mL] per serving)
> Each serving contains:
> Calories (Kcal): 2   Total fat (g): 0
> Carbohydrates (g): 1   Protein (g): 0
> Sodium (mg): 0   Cholesterol (mg): 0
> Diabetic exchange: free

Washington's Birthday Napoleon

For each napoleon prepare the following:

3 piles	phyllo dough napoleon rectangles (4 deep)	3 piles
¼ C	sugar-free vanilla pudding, made with skim milk	60 mL
2	maraschino cherries, finely chopped	2
1 t	fruit-only cherry preserves	5 mL
½ t	Cherry Glaze (p. 31)	3 mL

Bake sheets of phyllo according to the general instructions at the beginning of this chapter. Cut the pile of four sprayed sheets into 16 rectangles. Bake in a preheated 375°F (190°C) oven for 8 minutes. Three of these rectangular piles are used to make each napoleon.

Arrange one phyllo dough rectangle on a dessert plate. Put the vanilla pudding in a small bowl. Add the maraschino cherries. Mix well. Spread the cherry preserves gently onto the phyllo rectangle. Cover with a second rectangle. Pile the vanilla pudding on this layer. Spread to the edges. Put the last rectangle on top. Frost the top layer with Cherry Glaze.

Yield: 1 Washington's Birthday Napoleon
     Calories (Kcal): 86   Total fat (g): 0.9
     Carbohydrates (g): 16   Protein (g): 0.9
     Sodium (mg): 243   Cholesterol (mg): 1
     Diabetic exchange: 1 fruit

Cherry Glaze

This can be refrigerated and reheated when needed.

| ¼ C | sugar-free cherry preserves | 60 mL |
| 1 t | Kirsch wine (cherry liqueur) | 5 mL |

Put the cherry preserves into a small saucepan. Add the cherry liqueur and mix well with a fork or wire whisk. Heat gently, stirring constantly. Cool.

Yield: 12 servings
     Each serving contains:
     Calories (Kcal): 13   Total fat (g): 0
     Carbohydrates (g): 0   Protein (g): 0
     Sodium (mg): 3   Cholesterol (mg): 0
     Diabetic exchange: free

Mocha Napoleon

For each napoleon prepare the following:

3 piles	phyllo dough napoleon rectangles (4 deep)	3 piles
¼ C	Mocha Tart Filling (recipe follows)	60 mL
1 t	seedless, no-sugar-added raspberry jam	5 mL
¼ C	frozen low-fat non-dairy whipped topping	60 mL
1 t	Mocha Glaze (p. 33)	5 mL

Bake sheets of phyllo according to the general instructions at the beginning of this chapter. Cut the pile of four sprayed sheets into 16 rectangles. Bake in a preheated 375°F (190°C) oven for 8 minutes.

Arrange one phyllo rectangle on a dessert plate. Spread the Mocha Tart Filling on top of the phyllo. Put a second phyllo rectangle on a flat surface such as a tabletop. Carefully spread the raspberry jam on this rectangle and then place this, jam-side-up, on the previous layer. Spread the non-dairy whipped topping on top of the jam. Top this layer with the last rectangle. Smooth the Mocha Glaze on the top.

> Yield: 1 Mocha Napoleon
> Calories (Kcal): 122   Total fat (g): 3
> Carbohydrates (g): 18   Protein (g): 3
> Sodium (mg): 146   Cholesterol (mg): 1
> Diabetic exchange: 1 fruit; ½ high-fat meat

Mocha Tart Filling

For a sharper coffee taste, use instant espresso coffee powder.

1 pkg.(4 servings)	sugar-free chocolate pudding mix	1 pkg. (4 servings)
1½ C	skim milk	375 mL
3 t	instant coffee powder	15 mL

Combine all the ingredients in a saucepan. Bring to a boil and cook, stirring constantly until pudding has thickened.

> Yield: Enough for 6 napoleons
> The filling for each napoleon contains:
> Calories (Kcal): 24   Total fat (g): 0.1
> Carbohydrates (g): 4   Protein (g): 2
> Sodium (mg): 68   Cholesterol (mg): 1
> Diabetic exchange: 1 vegetable

Mocha Glaze

Drizzle over napoleons for a coffee-chocolate accent.

2 T	cocoa powder	30 mL
2 t	instant coffee powder	10 mL
2 T	hot water	30 mL
2 T	fat-free cream cheese	30 mL
2 t	aspartame sweetener	10 mL

Stir together the cocoa powder and instant coffee powder. Add the hot water and mix together until the mixture is smooth and evenly moist. Beat in the cream cheese and sweetener until smooth.

Yield: 15 servings
Each serving contains:

Calories (Kcal): 5	Total fat (g): 0.1
Carbohydrates (g): 0.9	Protein (g): 0.3
Sodium (mg): 9	Cholesterol (mg): 0
Diabetic exchange: free	

Banana Split Napoleon

For each napoleon, prepare the following:

3 piles	phyllo dough napoleon rectangles (4 deep)	3 piles
½ medium	ripe banana, peeled	½ medium
½ t	lemon juice	3 mL
2 T	sugar-free vanilla pudding made with skim milk	30 mL
2 t	crushed pineapple (packed in juice), drained	10 mL
2 T	frozen low-fat non-dairy whipped topping, thawed	30 mL
1 t	Chocolate Glaze (p. 35)	5 mL

Bake sheets of phyllo according to the general instructions at the beginning of this chapter. Cut the pile of four sprayed sheets into 16 rectangles. Bake in a preheated 375°F (190°C) oven for 8 minutes.

Arrange one phyllo rectangle on a dessert plate. Slice the banana into a bowl. Toss with the lemon juice and mash with a fork. Spread the banana evenly on the phyllo rectangle. Top with a second phyllo rectangle. Put the vanilla pudding in a small bowl. Add the pineapple and whipped topping. Blend with a fork and spread on top of the phyllo. Put the last rectangle onto a flat surface. Spread with the Chocolate Glaze gently, taking care not to break the phyllo. Top the napoleon with this layer.

Yield: 1 Banana Split Napoleon
 Calories (Kcal): 132 Total fat (g): 2
 Carbohydrates (g): 26 Protein (g): 2
 Sodium (mg): 159 Cholesterol (mg): 1
 Diabetic exchange: 1 fruit; 1 starch/bread

Chocolate Glaze

Add a little extra milk to get the right consistency if this is too thick.

2 T	cocoa powder	30 mL
2 T	skim milk	30 mL
2 T	fat-free cream cheese	30 mL
2 t	aspartame sweetener	10 mL

Combine the cocoa powder and skim milk in a small bowl until the mixture is moistened. Using a fork, beat in the cream cheese. The mixture will be smooth. Add in the aspartame and mix well.

> Yield: enough for 15 napoleons
> The filling for each napoleon contains:
> Calories (Kcal): 5   Total fat (g): 0.1
> Carbohydrates (g): 0.9   Protein (g): 0.4
> Sodium (mg): 10   Cholesterol (mg): 0
> Diabetic exchange: free

Hot Fudge Napoleon

For each napoleon, prepare the following:

3 piles	phyllo dough napoleon rectangles (4 deep)	3 piles
¼ C	sugar-free vanilla low-fat ice cream or frozen yogurt	60 mL
2 T	sugar-free vanilla pudding made with skim milk	30 mL
2 T	frozen low-fat non-dairy whipped topping, thawed	30 mL
5 t	Napoleon Fudge Topping (p. 37)	25 mL
1	fresh cherry or maraschino cherry	5 mL

Bake sheets of phyllo according to the general instructions at the beginning of this chapter. Cut the pile of four sprayed sheets into 16 rectangles. Bake in a preheated 375°F (190°C) oven for 8 minutes.

Arrange one phyllo rectangle on a dessert plate. Put the ice cream onto the rectangle and cover with another phyllo rectangle. In a small bowl, combine the pudding and whipped topping with a fork. Spread this onto the phyllo rectangle. Lay the last rectangle on the top of the pile. Top the napoleon with the hot Napoleon Fudge Topping and the cherry.

> Yield: 1 Hot Fudge Napoleon
> Calories (Kcal): 160   Total fat (g): 5
> Carbohydrates (g): 18   Protein (g): 3
> Sodium (mg): 260   Cholesterol (mg): 5
> Diabetic exchange: 1 starch/bread; 1 fat

Napoleon Fudge Topping

Rich and creamy, this topping tastes like the kind from the nicest bakeries.

2 T	cocoa powder, unsweetened	30 mL
1 t	canola oil	5 mL
2 t	skim milk	10 mL
2 t	aspartame sweetener	10 mL
½ t	vanilla extract	3 mL
1/8 t	butter extract	1 mL

Put the cocoa powder in a small saucepan. Add the canola oil and skim milk. Heat gently over a low flame, stirring constantly, until the mixture is blended and heated. Remove from heat. Stir in the aspartame and extracts and mix well. Spoon while still warm over the top of the napoleon.

Yield: enough for 2 napoleons
The topping for each napoleon contains:
Calories (Kcal): 90   Total fat (g): 3
Carbohydrates (g): 12   Protein (g): 2
Sodium (mg): 160   Cholesterol (mg): 0
Diabetic exchange: 1 starch/bread

Berry Good Napoleon

For each napoleon, prepare the following:

3 piles (4 deep)	phyllo dough napoleon rectangles	3 piles (4 deep)
2	fresh strawberries or frozen whole strawberries, defrosted, diced	2
6	fresh raspberries or frozen whole raspberries, defrosted, diced	6
2 T	lemon filling for Berry Good Napoleons (recipe follows)	30 mL
¼ C	sugar-free vanilla pudding made with skim milk	60 mL
2 T	frozen low-fat non-dairy whipped topping, thawed	30 mL

Bake sheets of phyllo according to the general instructions at the beginning of the chapter. Cut the pile of four sprayed sheets into 16 rectangles. Bake in a preheated 375°F (190°C) oven for 8 minutes.

Arrange one phyllo rectangle on a dessert plate. Mix the strawberries and raspberries together in a small bowl. Mash lightly with a fork. Set aside. Spread the lemon filling on the phyllo rectangle. Top with another rectangle. In another bowl, mix together the pudding and whipped topping. Do this gently with a fork. Spread the pudding on the rectangle. Top with the third rectangle. Spoon the fruit over the top.

> Yield: 1 Berry Good Napoleon
> Calories (Kcal): 102 Total fat (g): 2
> Carbohydrates (g): 17 Protein (g): 2
> Sodium (mg): 248 Cholesterol (mg): 0
> Diabetic exchange: 1 starch/bread

Lemon Filling for Berry Good Napoleon

Light and lemony.

1 T	cornstarch	15 mL
2 T	water	30 mL
⅓ C	fresh lemon juice	80 mL
7 pkgs.	acesulfame-K	7 pkgs.
¼ C	egg substitute	60 mL
2 t	vanilla extract	10 mL

Put the cornstarch and water into a small saucepan and mix to dissolve the cornstarch. Add the lemon juice and acesulfame-K. Cook gently, stirring constantly until the mixture thickens. In another pan, heat the egg substitute. Spoon some of the lemon mixture into the eggs. Mix well. Now combine in the rest of the lemon mixture and the vanilla extract. Cook over low heat for a minute or two. Cool.

Yield: 1 cup: enough for 8 Berry Good Napoleons
Filling for each napoleon contains:

Calories (Kcal): 14	Total fat (g): 0.3
Carbohydrates (g): 2	Protein (g): 0.1
Sodium (mg): 14	Cholesterol (mg): 0
Diabetic exchange: free	

Phyllo Strudel

You won't believe how easy strudel is until you try.

Read the directions for phyllo dough at the beginning of this chapter. Layer four sheets, spraying each from edge to edge with non-stick cooking spray. Don't cut them into napoleon rectangles. Leave one inch (2.5 cm) free of filling at each edge. Spoon the filling, leaving one inch (2.5 cm) clear from the left edge along the short side. Roll from the right side. The filling will roll up into the inside.

Put the roll on an ungreased cookie sheet with the seam down and tuck the ends under. Brush with melted butter. Bake in a preheated 325°F (165°C) oven for 25–30 minutes. Cool before slicing. Best if sliced with an electric knife or a very sharp serrated knife.

Yield: 10 slices
Each slice without the filling contains:

Calories (Kcal): 33	Total fat (g): 2
Carbohydrates (g): 4	Protein (g): 1
Sodium (mg): 48	Cholesterol (mg): 3
Diabetic exchange: ½ fat	

Cherry Strudel Filling

No one will believe this is low-calorie, it's so yummy.

1 lb	sweet cherries, pitted	450 g
¼ C	almonds, chopped	60 mL
2 T	sugar	30 mL

Combine all ingredients. Roll and bake in phyllo sheets as directed above.

Yield: filling for 10 servings
Filling for each serving contains:

Calories (Kcal): 63	Total fat (g): 2
Carbohydrates (g): 11	Protein (g): 1
Sodium (mg): 0	Cholesterol (mg): 0
Diabetic exchange: ½ starch/bread; ½ fat	

Apple Strudel Filling

The traditional filling you expect.

3	apples, peeled, cored, and sliced	3
¼ C	raisins	60 mL
¼ C	almonds, chopped	60 mL
2 T	sugar	30 mL
½ t	cinnamon	3 mL

Put the apples, raisins, and almonds in a mixing bowl. Toss to combine. In a small bowl, mix the sugar and cinnamon together. Toss with the apple mixture.

Roll and bake in phyllo sheets as directed on page 40.

Yield: filling for 10 servings
Filling for each serving contains:

Calories (Kcal): 66	Total fat (g): 2
Carbohydrates (g): 12	Protein (g): 0.9
Sodium (mg): 1	Cholesterol (mg): 0

Diabetic exchange: ½ fruit; ½ fat

Prune Filling for Strudel

When I make this strudel, everyone asks what the filling is made of. No one ever guesses prunes.

1 C	prunes, pitted	250 mL
½ C	unsweetened apple juice	125 mL
2 t	lemon peel	10 mL

In a small saucepan, cover the prunes with the juice. Bring to a boil over medium heat. Let stand 10 minutes. Pour off any unabsorbed liquid. Puree in a blender or food processor. Mix in the lemon peel. Roll and bake in phyllo sheets as directed on page 40.

Yield: filling for 10 servings
Each serving contains:

Calories (Kcal): 44	Total fat (g): 0.1
Carbohydrates (g): 11	Protein (g): 1
Sodium (mg): 1	Cholesterol (mg): 0

Diabetic exchange: ⅔ fruit

Apricot Filling for Strudel

A little sweet and tangy.

1 C	dried apricots	250 mL
½ C	orange juice	125 mL
2 t	orange rind	10 mL

Put the apricots into a small saucepan. Cover with orange juice. Bring to a boil. Let stand 10 minutes. Pour out any unabsorbed liquid. Puree in a food processor or blender. Mix in the orange rind. Roll and bake in phyllo sheets as directed on page 40.

> Yield: filling for 10 servings
> Each serving contains:
> Calories (Kcal): 44   Total fat (g): 0.1
> Carbohydrates (g): 11   Protein (g): 0.7
> Sodium (mg): 2   Cholesterol (mg): 0
> Diabetic exchange: ⅔ fruit

Phyllo Tarts

Handle phyllo sheets according to the general directions at the beginning of this chapter. Coat a 12-inch (30 cm) quiche or tart pan with non-stick cooking spray.

Prepare a stack of four sheets of phyllo dough, coating each layer evenly with non-stick cooking spray. Butter flavor is great! Using your pan as a pattern, cut a circle larger than the pan by enough extra so the dough will cover the sides of the pan.

Place the cut-out circle in the tart pan. Use your fingers to shape the dough to the bottom and sides of the pan. Brush with melted butter or margarine.

Bake the shell in a preheated 325°F (165°C) oven for 8–10 minutes. The shell will be lightly browned. Cool before filling. Remove from the pan and put it on a pretty dish or leave in the pan for extra strength.

Choose a filling found on the following pages, make it, and fill the shell.

Strawberry Cream Cheese Tart

Fat-free cream cheese makes this a low-calorie tart. It's very beautiful.

1	phyllo dough tart shell for 12" (30 cm) tart, baked	1
¼ C	sugar-free strawberry preserves	60 mL
1 T	water	15 mL
3 oz	fat-free cream cheese, softened	80 g pkg.
2 T	sugar	15 mL
2 T	cornstarch	15 mL
1 C	skim milk	250 mL
1 large	egg or equivalent egg substitute, lightly beaten	1 large
2 t	orange extract	5 mL
1 t	butter extract	5 mL
1 C	frozen low-fat non-dairy whipped topping, thawed	250 mL

Prepare the phyllo tart shell described on page 42. Mix together the strawberry preserves and water and spread carefully over the bottom of the tart shell. In a heavy-bottomed medium-size saucepan, combine the cream cheese, sugar, and cornstarch. Put over low heat and, stirring constantly, heat gently until the sugar is dissolved. Gradually stir in the milk and egg. When the mixture is smooth and combined, bring to a boil. Allow to bubble for one minute, stirring constantly. Cool, stirring occasionally. Stir in the extracts. Fold in the whipped topping. Refrigerate until completely cool. Spread the cream cheese mixture over the strawberry preserves.

Yield: 10 servings
Each serving contains:
Calories (Kcal): 88   Total fat (g): 2
Carbohydrates (g): 14   Protein (g): 2
Sodium (mg): 90   Cholesterol (mg): 23
Diabetic exchange: 1 starch/bread

Pistachio Pineapple Tart

A real treat for the eyes and taste buds.

1	phyllo dough tart shell for 12" (30 cm) tart, baked	1
1 pkg. (4 servings)	sugar-free pistachio no-cook pudding mix	1 pkg. (4 servings)
1¾ C	skim milk	435 mL
20 oz	pineapple slices, packed in juice, drained	565 g
8 t	fresh cherries, pitted	40 mL

Prepare the phyllo tart shell described on page 42. Put the phyllo shell on a dessert plate. Put the pudding mix into a medium mixing bowl. Add the milk and combine according to the directions on the package. Spoon into the tart shell. Dry the drained pineapple slices on paper towels. Arrange them on the pistachio pudding. Put the cherries in the center.

> Yield: 10 servings
> Each serving contains:
> Calories (Kcal): 105   Total fat (g): 0.6
> Carbohydrates (g): 24   Protein (g): 2
> Sodium (mg):   Cholesterol (mg): 1
> Diabetic exchange: 1 starch/bread; ½ fruit

Chocolate Tart Filling

You might want to use this plain, as an alternative to the chocolate-fruit combination.

¼ C	sugar	60 mL
3 pkgs.	acesufame-K or saccharin	3 pkgs.
2 T	cocoa powder, unsweetened	30 mL
3 T	cornstarch	45 mL
1¾ C	skim milk	435 mL
1 t	vanilla extract	5 mL
1 t	crème de cacao liqueur (optional)	5 mL

Combine the sugar, sugar substitute, cocoa powder, and cornstarch in a medium saucepan. Add a small amount of the milk. Stir with a wire whisk until the mixture is evenly moistened. Add the remainder of the milk, the vanilla extract, and the crème de cacao, if desired. Cook, stirring constantly until filling is thick and you can see whisk marks as you stir. Cool before pouring into tart shell. Makes 2 cups (500 mL).

> Yield: 10 servings
> Each serving contains:
> Calories (Kcal): 56   Total fat (g): 0.3
> Carbohydrates (g): 11   Protein (g): 2
> Sodium (mg): 54   Cholesterol (mg): 1
> Diabetic exchange: ⅔ starch/bread

Vanilla Tart Filling

This has the taste and consistency of a bakery tart filling. It's easy to prepare.

1¾ C	skim milk	435 mL
2 T	butter or margarine	30 mL
3 T	cornstarch	45 mL
2 T	sugar	30 mL
3 pkgs.	acesulfame-K	3 pkgs.
1 large	egg or equivalent egg substitute	1 large
1 T	vanilla extract	15 mL

Heat the milk and butter over simmering water in the top of a double boiler. In a bowl, mix together the cornstarch, sugar, and acesulfame-K. Add the egg and then the vanilla, blending well after each addition. Pour the cornstarch mixture into the warm milk. Mix with a wire whisk over simmering water until the mixture is thick. When the whisk leaves patterns, the pudding is finished cooking. Cool before using. Makes 2 cups (500 mL).

> Yield: 10 servings
> Each serving contains:
> Calories (Kcal): 63   Total fat (g): 3
> Carbohydrates (g): 7   Protein (g): 2
> Sodium (mg): 52   Cholesterol (mg): 28
> Diabetic exchange: ½ starch/bread; ½ fat

Chocolate Pear Tart

Since this uses canned pears, you can make it anytime.

1	phyllo dough tart shell for 12" (30 cm) tart, baked	1
2 C	Chocolate Tart Filling (it's very good with crème de cacao)	500 mL
15 oz	pear halves in water, no added sugar, drained	430 g

Prepare the phyllo tart shell described on page 42. Spoon the chocolate filling into the tart shell. Slice the pears thin (if this has not been done by the processor.) Put the slices onto paper towels to dry. Arrange the pears on the chocolate filling starting at the outside edge. Make a floral pattern in the center. This may be refrigerated for an hour before serving.

Yield: 10 servings
Each serving contains:
Calories (Kcal): 85   Total fat (g): 0.7
Carbohydrates (g): 17   Protein (g): 2
Sodium (mg): 82   Cholesterol (mg): 1
Diabetic exchange: 1 starch/bread

Chocolate Raspberry Tart

Chocolate and raspberry are a wonderful combination. You can make this all year round since the fresh raspberries are optional.

1	phyllo dough tart shell for 12" (30 cm) tart, baked	1
¼ C	seedless raspberry preserves, fruit only (no sugar added)	60 mL
2 C	Chocolate Tart Filling (pp. 44–45); (optional: add 2 T [30 mL] crème de cacao)	500 mL
½ C	frozen low-fat non-dairy whipped topping, thawed (optional)	125 mL
¼ C	fresh seedless raspberries (optional)	60 mL

Prepare the phyllo tart shell described on page 42. Smooth the raspberry preserves on the bottom of the inside of the tart shell. Spoon the chocolate filling on top of the preserves. Garnish with whipped topping and raspberries, if desired. May be refrigerated an hour or two before serving.

Yield: 10 servings
Each serving contains:

Calories (Kcal): 87	Total fat (g): 0.7
Carbohydrates (g): 18	Protein (g): 2
Sodium (mg): 82	Cholesterol (mg): 1

Diabetic exchange: 1 starch/bread

Banana Walnut Tart

A great solution for those ripe bananas.

1	phyllo dough tart shell for 12" (30 cm) tart, baked	1
¼ C	finely chopped walnuts	60 mL
2 C	Vanilla Tart Filling (p. 45)	500 mL
2 large	large ripe bananas	2 large
1 t	lemon juice	5 mL
3 pieces	mint leaves (optional)	3 pieces

Prepare the phyllo tart shell described on page 42. Mix the walnuts into the Vanilla Tart Filling before spooning it into the tart shell. Slice the bananas into a bowl. Add the lemon juice and, using a fork, toss gently to coat. Arrange the bananas in a spiral pattern on top of the filling. When you come around to the starting slice, move in one and repeat. A few mint leaves strategically placed in the center make a nice touch. May be refrigerated an hour or two before serving.

Yield: 10 servings
Each serving contains:

Calories (Kcal): 120	Total fat (g): 5
Carbohydrates (g): 16	Protein (g): 3
Sodium (mg): 80	Cholesterol (mg): 28

Diabetic exchange: 1 starch/bread; 1 fat

Tangerine Tart

A nice winter treat when tangerines are at their sweetest and cheapest!

1	phyllo dough tart shell for 12" (30 cm) tart, baked	1
2 C	Vanilla Tart Filling (p. 45), except use 1 t (5 mL) orange extract and 1 t (5 mL) vanilla extract instead of 1 T(15 mL) vanilla extract	500 mL
5	tangerines, peeled	5
5	cherries, pitted	5
2 T	shredded coconut meat (optional)	30 mL

Prepare the phyllo tart shell described on page 42. Spoon the Vanilla Tart Filling into the prepared shell. Remove any white strings or rind from the tangerine segments and separate the segments. Slice the inner skin carefully and slip out any seeds. Arrange the tangerine segments as spokes of wheels with a cherry in the center of each group on top of the tart filling. Sprinkle coconut over the top of the tangerine-and-cherry pattern. May be refrigerated an hour or two before serving.

> Yield: 10 servings
> Each serving contains:
> Calories (Kcal): 99   Total fat (g): 3
> Carbohydrates (g): 15   Protein (g): 2
> Sodium (mg): 80   Cholesterol (mg): 28
> Diabetic exchange: 1 starch/bread; ½ fat

Peach and Raspberry Tart

This is easy to create but looks fabulous. Try it when raspberries are in season.

1	phyllo dough tart shell for 12" (30 cm) tart, baked	1
2 C	Vanilla Tart Filling (p. 45); (optional: use Triple Sec instead of vanilla extract)	500 mL
15 oz	sliced peaches, packed without sugar in fruit juice	420 g can
1 C	fresh raspberries	250 mL

Prepare the phyllo tart shell described on page 42. Spoon the Vanilla Tart Filling into the tart shell. Drain the peaches and dry them on paper towels. Lay the peach slices on them flat-side-down, making a swirling pattern on the outside of the tart. Make a circle of raspberries inside. Then make a

flower of peach slices and raspberries in the center. May be refrigerated for
an hour before serving.

> Yield: 10 servings
> Each serving contains:
> Calories (Kcal): 88   Total fat (g): 3
> Carbohydrates (g): 13   Protein (g): 2
> Sodium (mg): 54   Cholesterol (mg): 28
> Diabetic exchange: 1 starch/bread; ½ fat

Strawberry-Kiwi Tart

A glorious end to a meal. Sonja's favorite, so we try to make it when she's coming to dinner.

1	phyllo dough tart shell for 12″ (30 cm) tart, baked (see p. 42)	1
2 C	Vanilla Tart Filling (p. 45)	500 mL
3 large	ripe kiwis, peeled and sliced	3 large
1 C	strawberries, hulled	250 mL

Prepare the phyllo tart shell as described on page 42. Spoon the Vanilla Tart
Filling into the prepared tart shell. Arrange the kiwi slices around the edge
of the tart. Stand a circle of strawberries inside the kiwi circle. Arrange the
remaining fruit on the inside of the tart. Serve immediately. This may be
refrigerated for an hour or two.

> Yield: 10 servings
> Each serving contains:
> Calories (Kcal): 98   Total fat (g): 4
> Carbohydrates (g): 14   Protein (g): 2
> Sodium (mg): 81   Cholesterol (mg): 28
> Diabetic exchange: 1 starch/bread; ½ fat

Orange Tart

If you use Triple Sec, it's very elegant.

1	baked phyllo dough tart shell for 12" (30 cm) tart	1
2 C	Vanilla Tart Filling (p. 45), except use 1 t (5 mL) or 2 t (10 mL) Triple Sec in place of the vanilla extract	500 mL
2	sweet oranges, peeled	2

Prepare the phyllo tart shell described on page 42. Spoon the tart filling into the tart shell. Pull any white strings off the oranges. With a sharp knife cut away any white areas. These will be bitter, so cut them away ruthlessly. Cut the orange crosswise into thin slices. Lay the slices in an overlapping pattern covering the entire surface of the tart. May be refrigerated for an hour or two before serving.

Yield: 10 servings
Each serving contains:
Calories (Kcal): 90   Total fat (g): 3
Carbohydrates (g): 14   Protein (g): 2
Sodium (mg): 80   Cholesterol (mg): 28
Diabetic exchange: 1 starch/bread; ½ fat

July 4th Tart

The red, white, and blue pattern is very patriotic. Sometimes we try to arrange the fruit in a flag design.

1	baked phyllo dough tart shell for 12" (30 cm) tart	1
2 C	Vanilla Tart Filling (p. 45)	500 mL
1 C	fresh blueberries	250 mL
1 C	fresh whole strawberries, hulled	250 mL

Prepare the phyllo tart shell described on page 42. Spoon the Vanilla Tart Filling into the prepared shell. Arrange the blueberries in a circle around the edge. Put the strawberries in a line across diagonally. Do this again to divide the tart into four sections. Arrange any remaining fruit in patterns in the open areas. May be refrigerated for an hour or two.

Yield: 10 servings
Each serving contains:

Calories (Kcal): 92   Total fat (g): 3
Carbohydrates (g): 13   Protein (g): 2
Sodium (mg): 81   Cholesterol (mg): 28
Diabetic exchange: 1 starch/bread; ½ fat

Pudding

Chocolate Mousse Pudding

Light and luscious. Meets a chocoholic's needs.

1½ C	skim milk	375 mL
1 pkg. (4 servings)	sugar-free, fat-free no-cook chocolate pudding mix	1 pkg. (4 servings)
1 C	frozen low-fat non-dairy whipped topping, thawed	250 mL
1 T	chocolate liqueur (optional) or crème de cacao (optional)	15 mL

Put the skim milk into a large mixing bowl. Add the pudding mix and beat one to two minutes. Add the whipped topping and chocolate liqueur or crème de cacao, if desired. Stir gently, until blended. Spoon into five dessert dishes.

Yield: 5 servings
Each serving contains:

Calories (Kcal): 37	Total fat (g): 2
Carbohydrates (g): 4	Protein (g) 0.6
Sodium (mg): 66	Cholesterol (mg): 2
Diabetic exchange: ½ fat	

Mocha Mousse Pudding

You'd never guess this is low in fat and calories.

1¾ C	skim milk	435 mL
¼ C	very strong brewed coffee	60 mL
1 pkg. (4 servings)	sugar-free, fat-free no-cook chocolate pudding mix	1 pkg. (4 servings)
1¼ C	frozen low-fat non-dairy whipped topping, thawed	310 mL
2 T	coffee liqueur	30 mL

Put the skim milk and coffee into a large mixing bowl. Add the pudding mix and beat one to two minutes. Add the whipped topping and coffee liqueur. Stir gently until blended. Spoon into five dessert dishes.

Yield: 5 servings
Each serving contains:
Calories (Kcal): 69   Total fat (g): 2
Carbohydrates (g): 8   Protein (g): 3
Sodium (mg): 67   Cholesterol (mg): 2
Diabetic exchange: ½ starch/bread; ½ fat

Quick (and Foolproof) Mocha Mousse

My cousin Ingrid couldn't believe how easy and impressive this was. I came up with the idea early one Sunday morning and we had it at breakfast.

1 pkg.	hot chocolate powder, no sugar added	1 pkg.
10 t	hot coffee	50 mL
2 C	frozen low-fat non-dairy whipped topping, thawed	500 mL

Put the hot chocolate powder into a medium mixing bowl. Add the coffee and stir until the powder is dissolved. Gently fold in the whipped topping until evenly mixed.

Yield: 4 servings
Each serving contains:
Calories (Kcal): 95   Total fat (g): 4
Carbohydrates (g): 11   Protein (g): 1
Sodium (mg): 40   Cholesterol (mg): 0
Diabetic exchange: 1 fruit; 1 fat

Thanksgiving Pumpkin Mousse

A light finish for a turkey dinner.

1¼ C	skim milk	310 mL
1 C	pumpkin pie filling	250 mL
¼ t	cinnamon	2 mL
¼ t	nutmeg	2 mL
¼ t	ginger	2 mL
1 pkg. (4 servings)	sugar-free no-cook butterscotch pudding mix	1 pkg. (4 servings)
1¼ C	water	310 mL
1 C	frozen low-fat non-dairy whipped topping	250 mL

In a mixing bowl, combine the milk, pumpkin, cinnamon, nutmeg, and ginger. Add the pudding mix and water and mix with a wire whisk or electric mixer until blended. Add the whipped topping and gently but thoroughly combine. Spoon into individual dessert dishes and chill 2–3 hours before serving.

Yield: 6 servings
Each serving contains:

Calories (Kcal): 101	Total fat (g): 2
Carbohydrates (g): 19	Protein (g): 3
Sodium (mg): 157	Cholesterol (mg): 1

Diabetic exchange: 1 starch/bread

Ricotta Cheese Pudding

A pudding for grown-ups—rich and very special.

1 lb	fat-free ricotta cheese	450 g
2 T	frozen low-fat non-dairy whipped topping	30 mL
2 T	Triple Sec	30 mL
1 t	aspartame sweetener	5 mL
2 oz	diabetic chocolate candy bar, coarsely chopped	55 g
¼ C	Not-Too-Sweet Chocolate Sauce (p. 55)	60 mL

Process the ricotta in a blender or food processor until smooth. Add the whipped topping, Triple Sec, and aspartame. Blend again. Transfer to a mixing bowl. Fold in the chocolate. Cover the bowl and refrigerate it for one hour before serving. Serve with chocolate sauce.

Yield: 4 servings
Each serving contains:
Calories (Kcal): 139   Total fat (g): 1
Carbohydrates (g): 16   Protein (g): 14
Sodium (mg): 88   Cholesterol (mg): 12
Diabetic exchange: 1½ milk

Not-Too-Sweet Chocolate Sauce

Stores well refrigerated, but warm gently before serving.

3 T	unsweetened cocoa powder	45 mL
1 T	flour	15 mL
1½ C	skim milk	375 mL
2 T	butter or margarine	30 mL
3 t	sugar substitute	15 mL
1 t	vanilla extract	5 mL
½ t	butter extract	3 mL

Combine the cocoa powder and flour in the top of a double boiler. Add the milk. Stir until free of lumps. Cook over boiling water, stirring until thick and smooth. Remove from heat. Stir in the butter. Cool for 15 minutes. Stir in the sugar substitute, vanilla extract, and butter extract. Serve over pudding or frozen treats.

Yield: 24 servings.
Each serving contains:
Calories (Kcal): 18   Total fat (g): 1
Carbohydrates (g): 2   Protein (g): 0.7
Sodium (mg): 19   Cholesterol (mg): 3
Diabetic exchange: free

Lemon Sponge Pudding

This is an adaptation of one of my Grandmother Lily's favorites.

1 T	flour	15 mL
2 T	sugar	30 mL
3 pkgs.	saccharin or acesulfame-K sugar substitute	3 pkgs.
2 T	lemon juice	30 mL
1½ t	lemon peel	8 mL
2 large	eggs, separated	2 large
1 C	skim milk	250 mL

In a mixing bowl, combine flour, sugar, sugar substitute, lemon juice, and lemon peel. Mix. In another bowl, beat the egg yolks at high speed until lemon colored. Add the yolks to the flour mixture. Blend well. Beat the egg whites until stiff. Fold them into the custard mixture. Pour the pudding into a casserole coated with non-stick cooking spray. Put the casserole in a pan of hot water in a preheated 350°F (180°C) oven. Bake for 35–40 minutes. The top will be lightly browned.

> Yield: 4 servings
> Each serving contains:
> Calories (Kcal): 95   Total fat (g): 3
> Carbohydrates (g): 12   Protein (g): 6
> Sodium (mg): 66   Cholesterol (mg): 107
> Diabetic exchange: 1 milk

Quick (Microwave) Custard

When I first made this I couldn't believe how quick custard could be.

1½ C	skim milk	375 mL
3 large	eggs, or equivalent egg substitute	3 large
2 T	sugar	30 mL
3 pkgs.	saccharin	3 pkgs.
1 t	vanilla	5 mL
¼ t	nutmeg	2 mL

Pour the milk into a glass measuring cup and put it in the microwave on high for three minutes. In a mixing bowl, stir together the eggs, sugar, sugar substitute, and vanilla. Gradually stir in the hot milk. Pour into a glass baking dish. Sprinkle nutmeg on top. Cook on "defrost" in the microwave for 10 minutes. The custard will become more firm as it sets.

Yield: 4 servings
Each serving contains:

Calories (Kcal): 117	Total fat (g): 4
Carbohydrates (g): 12	Protein (g): 8
Sodium (mg): 98	Cholesterol (mg): 161

Diabetic exchange: 1 milk; ½ fat

Microwave Vanilla Pudding

Perfect for a lazy-day dessert. A spoonful of Not-Too-Sweet Chocolate Sauce makes it extra special.

3 T	sugar	45 mL
2 T	cornstarch	30 mL
2 C	skim milk	500 mL
1 large	egg or equivalent egg substitute	1 large
1 t	butter or margarine	5 mL
2 t	vanilla	10 mL
2 pkgs.	sugar substitute	2 pkgs.

Put the sugar and cornstarch in a 4-cup (1 L) glass mixing bowl. Mix in the skim milk. Cook on "high" in the microwave for 5–7 minutes. Stop a few times to stir during the process. The mixture will be smooth and thick. Beat the egg in a small bowl. Mix in a few spoonfuls of the hot milk mixture. Turn the egg mixture into the thickened milk. Mix well. Return to the microwave and cook on "roast" or "medium" for a minute or two. Stop and stir during the process. Remove from the microwave. Stir in the butter, vanilla, and sugar substitute.

Yield: 4 servings
Each serving contains:

Calories (Kcal): 126	Total fat (g): 2
Carbohydrates (g): 20	Protein (g): 6
Sodium (mg): 91	Cholesterol (mg): 58

Diabetic exchange: 1 starch/bread; ½ milk

Banana Pudding

Elvis' favorite!

4 large	eggs	4 large
¼ C	sugar	60 mL
3 T	flour	45 mL
2 C	skim milk	250 mL
1 t	vanilla	5 mL
18	vanilla wafers	18
4 medium	bananas, ripe, peeled and sliced	4 medium
1 T	sugar	15 mL

Separate 3 eggs. Put the 3 yolks and the remaining whole egg in the top of a double boiler. Add the sugar and mix well. Stir in the flour. Using a wire whisk, stir in the milk. Put the top of the double boiler over boiling water and cook, stirring constantly until the mixture thickens. Stir in the vanilla and cool slightly. Spoon some custard onto the bottom of a 10-cup (1.5 L) casserole. Form a layer on top of the custard using 6 wafers. Cover with a layer of banana slices. Repeat layerings, ending with custard. Beat the egg whites and remaining sugar until stiff. Spoon this meringue on top of the pudding. Cover entirely, up to the edges. (If the meringue doesn't attach to the edges it will shrink during baking.) Bake in a preheated 425°F (220°C) oven for about five minutes. The meringue will be delicately browned.

Yield: 8 servings
Each serving contains:
Calories (Kcal): 216   Total fat (g): 5
Carbohydrates (g): 36   Protein (g): 7
Sodium (mg): 105   Cholesterol (mg): 107
Diabetic exchange: 2 starch/bread; 1 fat

Roll-Ups

Walnut Roll-Up Cookies

Most diabetic diet cookies are pretty inedible, in my opinion. These are the exceptions.

1 pkg.	active dry yeast	1 pkg.
¼ C	warm water	60 mL
2 C	flour	500 mL
¼ C+2 T	fat-free fruit-based butter-and-oil replacement	90 mL
2 T	oil replacement	30 mL
1 large	egg or equivalent egg substitute, lightly beaten	1 large
3 oz	fat-free cream cheese	80 g
2 T	sugar	15 mL
1 t	orange peel, grated	5 mL
1 t	orange extract	5 mL
½ C	walnuts, finely ground	125 mL

In a small mixing bowl, combine the yeast and warm water. In a large mixing bowl, combine the flour and butter replacement. Beat in the egg. Add the yeast and mix just until blended. On a lightly floured board, roll out the dough into two 13 × 9" (33 × 22 cm) rectangles. In a mixing bowl, beat the cream cheese until light and fluffy. Add the sugar, orange peel, and the orange extract. Beat well. Spread half the cream cheese mixture on each rectangle. Sprinkle with walnuts. Starting at the long side, roll up the rectangles. Place each roll on a cookie sheet that has been coated with non-stick vegetable cooking spray. Put the seam side down. Bake in a preheated 375°F (190°C) oven for 20–25 minutes. Cool. Cut into 1-inch (2.5 cm) slices.

> Yield: 24 cookies
> Each cookie contains:
> Calories (Kcal): 73   Total fat (g): 2
> Carbohydrates (g): 12   Protein (g): 3
> Sodium (mg): 14   Cholesterol (mg): 9
> Diabetic exchange: 1 starch/bread

Sweet Crêpe Batter

If the first crêpe doesn't move easily in the pan, blend in a little additional milk.

2 large	eggs, or equivalent egg substitute	2 large
3 T	canola oil	45 mL
1 t	butter extract	5 mL
1 C	skim milk	250 mL
2 T	fruit-flavored liqueur	30 mL
½ C	flour	125 mL
1 T	sugar	15 mL

Put the ingredients in the blender or food processor in the order listed. Blend at high speed for a minute or more, until the batter is well blended. Cover and refrigerate for an hour or more. To prepare the crêpes, coat a medium-sized heavy-bottomed frying pan with butter-flavored vegetable cooking spray. Heat the pan until it is hot. Remove the pan from the heat source and pour ¼ cup (60 mL) of the batter into the center of the pan. Tilt the pan quickly in all directions to coat the bottom. Return the pan to the heat and cook for a minute or so. Shake the pan to loosen the crêpe. Lift one edge of the crêpe. If it's a light, golden color it's done. Turn the crêpe with a spatula and brown this side for about 30 seconds. This side won't look as good and should become the inside when you wrap the crêpes around the filling.

Yield: 6 crêpes
Each crêpe contains:

Calories (Kcal): 80	Total fat (g): 4
Carbohydrates (g): 6	Protein (g): 2
Sodium (mg): 21	Cholesterol (mg): 36

Diabetic exchange: ½ starch/bread; 1 fat

Blintz Filling for Crêpes

The butter extract gives this filling a rich flavor.

1 lb	fat-free cottage cheese	450 g
2 pkgs.	sugar substitute	2 pkgs.
1 t	butter extract	5 mL
2 T	frozen low-fat non-dairy whipped topping	30 mL

Put all the ingredients into a blender or food processor. Blend until smooth. To serve, put a spoonful of the mixture on the last-cooked side of the crêpe.

Yield: Filling for 6 crêpes
Each crêpe filling includes:
Calories (Kcal): 49   Total fat (g): 0.2
Carbohydrates (g): 5   Protein (g): 9
Sodium (mg): 202   Cholesterol (mg): 7
Diabetic exchange: 1 lean meat

Austrian Raspberry Cream Crêpes

You'll think you're in Vienna.

1 recipe	Sweet Crêpe Batter	1 recipe
1 C	fruit-only seedless raspberry preserves	250 mL
½ C	water	125 mL
2 T	raspberry flavored brandy (optional)	30 mL
1½ C	fat-free sour cream	375 mL
⅓ C	toasted almonds, finely chopped (optional)	80 mL

Prepare the crêpes according to the directions (p. 60). Put waxed paper between them as you prepare them and a towel over the top to keep them warm. In a small saucepan, mix together the preserves, water, and brandy, if you are using it. Heat for 5 minutes or so, stirring constantly. Remove from heat. In a small mixing bowl, mix together the sour cream and almonds, if desired. Spread 2 T (30 mL) of the raspberry mixture on the back of each crêpe, and roll it with the raspberry inside. Arrange crêpes on dessert plates. Spoon on a dollop of sour cream and garnish with any remaining raspberry mixture.

Yield: 12 servings
Each serving contains:
Calories(Kcal)   148 Total fat (g): 4
Carbohydrates (g): 21   Protein (g): 3
Sodium (mg): 46   Cholesterol (mg): 36
Diabetic exchange: 1 starch/bread; ½ fruit; 1 fat

Kaiser Schmarren

An old German recipe.

1 recipe	Sweet Crêpe Batter (p. 60)	1 recipe
½ C	orange juice	125 mL
1 t	orange extract	5 mL
½ C	raisins (golden are prettiest)	125 mL
1 t	butter or margarine	5 mL
½ C	almonds, sliced	125 mL

Prepare the crêpes according to the general directions. In a small bowl, mix together the orange juice, orange extract, and raisins. Let stand for half an hour or so, until the raisins are plump. Melt the butter in a small frying pan. Add the almonds and toast them until they are golden, stirring constantly. Combine the raisin and almond mixtures. Distribute inside each crêpe before rolling.

Yield: 12 servings
Each serving contains:

Calories (Kcal): 68	Total fat (g): 4
Carbohydrates (g): 8	Protein (g): 2
Sodium (mg): 6	Cholesterol (mg): 4

Diabetic exchange: ½ starch/bread; ½ fat

Crêpes Marcelles

Roll these just before serving. I've used instant pudding in a pinch in place of the tart filling.

1 recipe	Sweet Crêpe Batter (p. 60)	1 recipe
1 recipe	Vanilla Tart Filling (p. 45)	1 recipe
1 T	cognac	15 mL
1 t	orange extract	5 mL
¼ C	crushed pineapple in juice, drained	60 mL

Prepare the crêpes according to the general directions. Prepare the Vanilla Tart Filling. Mix in the cognac, orange extract, and crushed pineapple. Spoon this filling into the crêpes and roll them before serving.

Yield: 12 servings
Each serving contains:
Calories (Kcal): 64   Total fat (g): 3
Carbohydrates (g): 7   Protein (g): 2
Sodium (mg): 45   Cholesterol (mg): 26
Diabetic exchange: ½ starch/bread; ½ fat

Basic Roll-Up Recipe

Use this for all the "jelly roll" style recipes that follow. It's easy to do.

1 C	cake flour, sifted	250 mL
1 t	baking powder	5 mL
3 large	eggs	3 large
¼ C	sugar	60 mL
3 pkgs.	acesulfame-K	3 pkgs.
⅓ C	water	80 mL
1 t	vanilla extract	5 mL

Spray a 15×10×1" (37×25×3 cm) jelly-roll pan; line the bottom with waxed paper; spray the paper. Sift the flour and baking powder together. With an electric mixer, beat the eggs in a medium bowl until thick and creamy and light in color. Gradually add the sugar and the acesulfame-K, beating constantly until the mixture is very thick. Stir in the water and vanilla. Fold in the flour mixture. Spread the batter evenly in the prepared pan.

Bake at 375°F (190°C) for 12 minutes or until the center of the cake springs back when lightly pressed. Loosen the cake around the edges with a knife. Invert the pan onto a clear tea towel, and peel off the waxed paper. Starting at the short end, roll up the cake and towel together. Place the roll seam-side-down on a wire rack and cool completely. When cool unroll carefully and assemble with filling. With a sharp knife, score the places where the slices will be, so they are even.

Yield: 10 servings
Each serving contains:

Calories (Kcal): 82	Total fat (g): 2
Carbohydrates (g): 14	Protein (g): 3
Sodium (mg): 56	Cholesterol (mg): 64
Diabetic exchange: 1 starch/bread	

Fresh Strawberry Roll-Up

Annette says this is her new substitute for strawberry shortcake. She loved it for dessert at her Fourth of July cookout.

1 recipe	Basic Roll-Up Recipe (above)	1 recipe
2 C	frozen low-fat non-dairy whipped topping	500 mL
2 C	fresh strawberries, hulled and quartered	500 mL

Prepare the Basic Roll-Up Recipe. Cool and unroll. Stir the non-dairy whipped topping and the strawberries together. Spread this filling evenly on the roll. Starting from the short end, roll up the cake by lifting the cake with the end of the towel. Place the roll seam-side-down on a serving plate.

Yield: 10 slices
Each serving contains:

Calories (Kcal): 124	Total fat (g): 4
Carbohydrates (g): 19	Protein (g): 3
Sodium (mg): 56	Cholesterol (mg): 64

Diabetic exchange: 1 starch/bread; 1 fat

Chocolate Roll-Up

If you love chocolate this will be your favorite.

1 recipe	Basic Roll-Up Recipe (p. 64)	1 recipe
1 pkg. (4 servings)	sugar-free low-fat no-cook chocolate pudding mix	1 pkg. (4 servings)
1½ C	skim milk	375 mL
2 T	crème de cacao (optional)	30 mL
½ C	white topping (optional)	125 mL

Prepare the Basic Roll-Up Recipe. Cool and unroll. Put the pudding mix in a mixing bowl. Add the skim milk and crème de cacao, if desired. Whip until thickened. Spread the pudding on the roll. Roll up the cake from the short end. To start rolling, lift the cake with the end of the towel. When rolled, place the roll seam-side-down on a serving plate. Optional: Top each slice with a dollop of your favorite white topping.

Yield: 10 slices
Each slice contains:

Calories (Kcal): 96	Total fat (g): 2
Carbohydrates (g): 17	Protein (g): 5
Sodium (mg): 97	Cholesterol (mg): 65

Diabetic exchange: 1 fruit; ½ lean meat

Peach Melba Roll-Up

Since there is no fresh fruit, you can make this "off the shelf" anytime.

1 recipe	Basic Roll-Up Recipe (p. 64)	1 recipe
1 recipe	Vanilla Tart Filling (p. 45)	1 recipe
15 oz	sliced peaches in juice, drained	425 g can

Prepare the Basic Roll-Up Recipe. Cool and unroll. Prepare the tart filling and then spread it evenly on the cooled roll. Arrange the peach slices all over the surface and roll up the cake from the short end. To start rolling, lift the cake with the end of the towel. When rolled, place the roll seam-side-down on a serving plate.

> Yield: 10 slices
> Each slice contains:
> Calories (Kcal): 164   Total fat (g): 5
> Carbohydrates (g): 26   Protein (g): 5
> Sodium (mg): 110   Cholesterol (mg): 92
> Diabetic exchange: 1½ starch/bread; ½ fat

Banana Walnut Roll-Up

Annette's brother Mark, from Philadelphia, loved this one!

1 recipe	Basic Roll-Up Recipe (p. 64)	1 recipe
1 recipe	Vanilla Tart Filling (p. 45)	1 recipe
3 small	ripe bananas, peeled and sliced	3 small
¼ C	chopped walnuts	60 mL

Prepare the Basic Roll-Up Recipe. Cool and unroll. Prepare the tart filling and then stir the bananas and walnuts into it. Spread the filling evenly on the cooked roll and roll up the cake from the short end. To start rolling, lift the cake with the end of the towel. When rolled, place the roll seam-side-down on a serving plate.

> Yield: 10 slices
> Each slice contains:
> Calories (Kcal): 195   Total fat (g): 7
> Carbohydrates (g): 29   Protein (g): 6
> Sodium (mg): 108   Cholesterol (mg): 92
> Diabetic exchange: 2 starch/bread; 1 fat

Mocha Raspberry Roll-Up

A grown-up taste. Very elegant.

1 recipe	Basic Roll-Up Recipe (p. 64)	1 recipe
1 recipe	Mocha Tart Filling (p. 32)	1 recipe
2 C	fresh raspberries	500 mL

Prepare the Basic Roll-Up Recipe. Cool and unroll. Prepare the tart filling, spread it evenly on the cooled roll, and sprinkle the raspberries all over the surface. Roll up the cake from the short end. To start rolling, lift the cake with the end of the towel. When rolled, place the roll seam-side-down on a serving plate.

Yield: 10 slices
Each slice contains:
Calories (Kcal): 96   Total fat (g): 2
Carbohydrates (g): 17   Protein (g): 3
Sodium (mg): 63   Cholesterol (mg): 64
Diabetic exchange: 1 starch/bread; ½ fat

Pistachio Pineapple Roll-Up

The pineapple adds a lightness to the pistachio pudding mix.

1 recipe	Basic Roll-Up Recipe (p. 64)	1 recipe
1 pkg. (4 servings)	sugar-free instant pistachio pudding mix	1 pkg. (4 servings)
1¾ C	skim milk	435 mL
1 C	crushed pineapple in juice, drained	250 mL

Prepare the Basic Roll-Up Recipe. Cool and unroll. Put the pudding mix into a mixing bowl. Add the skim milk and mix until the pudding is thick. Beat in the pineapple. Spread this filling evenly on the roll and roll up the cake, starting from the short end. To start the rolling, lift the cake with the end of the towel. Place the roll seam-side-down on a serving plate.

Yield: 10 slices
Each slice contains:
Calories (Kcal): 114   Total fat (g): 2
Carbohydrates (g): 21   Protein (g): 5
Sodium (mg): 100   Cholesterol (mg): 65
Diabetic exchange: 1½ fruit; ½ fat

Apricot Roll-Up

You don't need to know anything about baking to do a great job with this.

1 recipe	Basic Roll-Up Recipe (p. 64)	1 recipe
½ C	fruit-only apricot preserves	125 mL
¼ C	water	60 mL

Prepare the Basic Roll-Up Recipe. Cool and unroll. In a small saucepan, mix together the preserves and water over low heat. The heat will help the blending process. Spread the apricot mixture evenly on the roll and roll up the cake, starting from the short end. To start the rolling, lift the cake with the end of the towel. Place the roll seam-side-down on a serving plate

Yield: 10 slices
Each slice contains:
Calories (Kcal): 111   Total fat (g): 2
Carbohydrates (g): 21   Protein (g): 3
Sodium (mg): 56   Cholesterol (mg): 64
Diabetic exchange: 1 starch/ bread; ½ fat

Meringues

Meringues

The recipes in this chapter are all based on meringue—beaten egg whites slowly baked. They are low in fat and very elegant. You might think meringues are beyond your capabilities—they are not! It's hard to go wrong if you follow a few simple rules.

•Don't use plastic when you beat the egg whites. Glass or metal bowls give the most fluff from egg whites.

•Be sure your utensils are spotless. For egg whites to beat up, the bowls, blades, and scrapers should be grease-free.

•Be sure no bits of yolk are mixed in with the whites. Separate whites and yolks into small cups or bowls, and put only pure egg whites into the mixing bowl. Should the yolk bread during the separation process, put that egg aside and use another one.

•Don't bake meringues on wax paper or plain cookie sheets. Use parchment paper or the inside of clean brown paper grocery bags.

•Recognize that humidity changes meringues. On high-humidity days, meringues are chewy. On low-humidity days, meringues are dry and crispy.

•Never open the oven, even to peek, until the stated time has elapsed.

•Use reconstituted "Just Whites" powdered egg whites if you have no use for leftover yolks. They may be found in your supermarket, health food store, or gourmet shop.

•Even though egg substitutes are mostly egg whites, they don't work for meringues.

•Freeze meringues after you've made them or store them at room temperature. Always keep meringues in airtight containers.

Basic Meringue

Follow the meringue advice for best results.

3 large	egg whites	3 large	
¼ t	cream of tartar	2 mL	
¼ C	sugar	60 mL	

Preheat the oven to 250°F (120°C) or the temperature specified in the specific recipe. Cut a brown paper grocery bag or parchment paper to the same size as your cookie sheet. Place the paper on top of the cookie sheet. Using plates, cups, or saucers and a pencil, trace the shape specified in the recipe onto the paper. In a large glass or metal bowl, beat the egg whites with the cream of tartar using an electric mixer. When soft peaks begin to form, keep beating, but slowly add the sugar. Increase the mixer speed until stiff peaks form and the meringue is glossy. Don't beat past this point or the meringue will become too dry!

With a clean spoon or rubber scraper transfer the beaten egg white to the circles drawn on the paper. Bake in a 250°F (120°C) preheated oven for the amount of time specified in the recipe. When the time is up, turn off the oven but don't open the oven door. Leave the meringues in the turned-off oven for two more hours. Then carefully remove the cookie sheets from the oven. Use a spatula to loosen the meringue from the paper.

Yield: 1 Basic Meringue recipe (4 servings)

Each serving contains:
Calories (Kcal): 61   Total fat (g): 0
Carbohydrates (g): 13   Protein (g): 3
Sodium (mg): 41   Cholesterol (mg): 0
Diabetic exchange: 1 starch/bread

Lime Kisses

Anna and Adie call these "Surprise Kisses" because of the sparkly sensation you get in your mouth. They love them!

1 recipe	Basic Meringue (above)	1 recipe	
1 pkg.	sugar-free lime gelatin powder	four servings	

Prepare the Basic Meringue, but add the lime gelatin along with the sugar. Use a brown paper bag or parchment paper to cover an ungreased cookie sheet. Drop the meringue by teaspoonfuls (5 mL) onto the cookie sheet.

Put the kisses into a preheated 275°F (135°C) oven for 30 minutes. Turn off the oven. Keep the kisses in the oven for another 10 minutes without opening the door. Use a spatula to remove the kisses from the paper.

> Yield: 5 dozen Lime Kisses
> Each kiss contains:
> Calories (Kcal): 4   Total fat (g): 0
> Carbohydrates (g): 1   Protein (g): 0.2
> Sodium (mg): 6   Cholesterol (mg): 0
> Diabetic exchange: free

Tart Orange Meringue Tarts

Thin slices of orange make a festive garnish.

1 recipe	Basic Meringue (p. 70)	1 recipe
2 T	sugar	30 mL
4 t	cornstarch	20 mL
1 C	unsweetened orange juice	250 mL
1 T	lemon juice (fresh is best)	15 mL
1 t	aspartame sweetener	5 mL
½ C	white topping (optional)	125 mL

Prepare the Basic Meringue with the following variation: Draw six 4" (10 cm) circles on the brown paper. Spoon the meringue into the circles, building up the edges by an inch (2.5 cm), and form a depression in the middle to make a tart shell. Bake in a preheated 250°F (120°C) oven for 1 hour. Cool in the oven for two hours longer without opening the door.

After the meringues are in the oven, prepare the filling by combining the sugar and cornstarch in a saucepan. Use a whisk to blend in the orange juice. Stirring constantly, cook over a medium heat until mixture thickens. Remove from heat and stir in the orange juice, lemon juice, and aspartame. Cool and store in the refrigerator until just before serving. Then, spoon the filling into the cooked meringue shells. Top with a dollop of your favorite white topping, if desired.

> Yield: 6 Orange Meringue Tarts
> Each tart contains:
> Calories (Kcal): 84   Total fat (g): 0.1
> Carbohydrates (g): 19   Protein (g): 2
> Sodium (mg): 28   Cholesterol (mg): 0
> Diabetic exchange: 1 starch/bread

Valentine Tarts

Prepare these for your honey any day of the year, but I like them in heart shapes for Valentine's Day.

1 recipe	Basic Meringue (p. 70)	1 recipe
1 lb	sweet cherries, pitted	450 g
1 T	sugar	15 mL
1 T	brandy or water	15 mL

Prepare the meringue according to the directions for Basic Meringue. Trace eight circles or hearts about 2½" (12 cm) in diameter onto parchment or onto the inside of clean brown paper grocery bags cut to the size of your cookie sheets. Spoon the meringue inside the patterns and smooth to the shapes traced. Place in a preheated 250°F (120°C)oven for 30 minutes. Leave the oven door closed, turn off the heat, and let the meringue remain in the oven for two more hours. Cool on a wire rack.

Using a spatula, carefully remove the meringues from the paper. Place one meringue on each of four dessert plates. Prepare the cherry topping by putting the cherries, sugar, and brandy or water in a microwave-safe bowl. Stir. Microwave for a minute or two on "high" until the cherries become juicy and steamy. Alternatively, put the cherries, sugar, and brandy or water into a medium saucepan. Stir constantly and heat until the berries are soft and juicy. Put a spoonful of the sauce on top of each of the four meringues. Top each with a second meringue and then distribute the remaining cherries. Top with a dollop of your favorite white topping, if desired.

Yield: 4 Valentine Tarts
Each tart contains:
Calories (Kcal): 164   Total fat (g): 1
Carbohydrates (g): 35   Protein (g): 4
Sodium (mg): 41   Cholesterol (mg): 0
Diabetic exchange: 1 starch/bread; 1½ fruit

Tangerine Cream Tarts

Great in the winter when tangerines are sweet.

1 recipe	Basic Meringue (p. 70)	1 recipe
8 oz	fat-free cream cheese	225 g
3 T	Triple Sec	45 mL
4 t	cornstarch	20 mL
1⅓ C	orange or tangerine juice, unsweetened (okay from frozen concentrate)	330 mL
3	tangerines, peeled and separated into segments, pitted	3

Prepare the Basic Meringue. To prepare the filling, put the cream cheese in a mixing bowl. Add the liqueur and beat until well mixed. Put the cornstarch into a small saucepan. Stir in the orange juice very gradually. Bring to a boil, stirring constantly. Boil for one minute. Remove from heat. Snip the center of each tangerine segment and remove the seeds. Put the seedless tangerine segments into the saucepan with the thickened juice. Put one-sixth of the cheese filling into the bottom of each meringue shell. Top with one-sixth of the tangerine mixture. Chill 1–2 hours before serving.

Yield: 6 Tangerine Cream Tarts
Each tart contains:
Calories (Kcal): 151   Total fat (g): 0.2
Carbohydrates (g): 26   Protein (g): 5
Sodium (mg): 209   Cholesterol (mg): 7
Diabetic exchange: 2 starch/bread

Traditional Pavlova

This lovely dessert was created for the graceful Anna Pavlova, the Russian ballerina who visited New Zealand and Australia in the early 1900s.

1 recipe	Basic Meringue (p. 70)	1 recipe
2 C	frozen low-fat non-dairy whipped topping, thawed	500 mL
2 C	fresh strawberries, hulled	500 mL
4	ripe kiwi fruit, peeled	4

Prepare the Basic Meringue. Trace a 12" (30 cm) circle on the inside of a clean brown paper grocery bag or a piece of parchment paper. Put the paper on an ungreased cookie sheet. Spoon the meringue into the circle. Spread so it is evenly distributed. Bake in a preheated 250°F (120°C) oven for 1 hour. Turn off the oven. Leave the meringue in the oven for an additional 30 minutes without opening the door. Then cool on a wire rack. Carefully remove the brown paper and place the meringue on a serving plate. Just before serving, spread the whipped topping carefully over the top of the meringue. Slice the strawberries lengthwise. Place them, cut-side-down, so the points extend out past the edge of the meringue. Slice the kiwis in thin "coins" and overlap them in a ring. Arrange the remaining strawberries in the center.

> Yield: 10 servings
> Each serving contains:
> Calories (Kcal): 84   Total fat (g): 2
> Carbohydrates (g): 15   Protein (g): 2
> Sodium (mg): 18   Cholesterol (mg): 0
> Diabetic exchange: 1 starch/bread

Pavlova Wedges with Kiwis and Raspberry Sauce

Individual servings of a variation of the traditional Pavlova.

1 recipe	Basic Meringue (p. 70)	1 recipe
4	ripe kiwis	4
1 recipe	Raspberry Sauce (recipe follows)	1 recipe

Prepare the Basic Meringue. Trace a 12" (30 cm) circle on the inside of a clean brown paper grocery bag or a piece of parchment paper. Put the paper on an ungreased cookie sheet. Spoon the meringue into the circle. Spread the meringue so it is evenly distributed. Bake in a preheated 250°F (120°C) oven for 1 hour. Turn off the oven. Leave the meringue in the oven for an additional 30 minutes without opening the door. Carefully cut the meringue into eight wedges. Put each wedge on a dessert plate. Peel the kiwis. Slice thinly. Arrange one-half sliced kiwi on each slice of meringue. Spoon raspberry sauce over the fruit and meringue.

Yield: 8 servings
Each serving contains:

Calories (Kcal): 98	Total fat (g): 0.2
Carbohydrates (g): 21	Protein (g): 2
Sodium (mg): 31	Cholesterol (mg): 0

Diabetic exchange: 1 starch/bread; ½ fruit

Raspberry Sauce

Seedless raspberry preserves are the best and are worth hunting down.

½ C	no-sugar-added seedless raspberry preserves	125 mL
2 T	Chambord liqueur or raspberry brandy	30 mL
2 T	water	30 mL

Put the preserves into a small saucepan. Add the raspberry liqueur and water. Mix well with a wire whisk. Heat gently, stirring constantly.

Yield: ¾ cup (185 mL) or 8 servings
One recipe of Raspberry Sauce contains:

Calories (Kcal): 44	Total fat (g): 0
Carbohydrates (g): 9	Protein (g): 0
Sodium (mg): 7	Cholesterol (mg): 0

Diabetic exchange: ½ fruit

French Raspberry Pavlova

You will be a hit with everyone when you serve this. Don't expect leftovers!

1 recipe	Basic Meringue (p. 70)	1 recipe
1 recipe	Vanilla Tart Filling (p. 45)	1 recipe
2 C	fresh raspberries	500 mL

Prepare the Basic Meringue. Trace a 12" (30 cm) circle on the inside of a clean brown paper grocery bag or a piece of parchment paper cut to fit your cookie sheet. Put the paper on an ungreased cookie sheet. Spoon the meringue into the circle. Spread so it is evenly distributed. Bake in a preheated 250°F (120°F) oven for 1 hour. Turn off the oven. Don't open the door. Leave the meringue in the oven for an additional 30 minutes. Remove to a wire rack to cool.

Carefully separate the meringue from the paper using a spatula. Place the meringue on a serving plate. Prepare the Vanilla Tart Filling. Spoon on the filling. Smooth it evenly to the edges. Arrange the raspberries in concentric circles, beginning at the outside edge. Serve immediately. Meringue gets soggy in damp weather and as the filling sits on top of it. Nevertheless, my family loves the refrigerated leftovers for breakfast!

Yield: 10 servings
Each serving contains:

Calories (Kcal): 100	Total fat (g): 3
Carbohydrates (g): 15	Protein (g): 3
Sodium (mg): 69	Cholesterol (mg): 28

Diabetic exchange: 1 starch/bread; ½ fat

Peach Pavlova

This Pavlova uses ice cream or frozen yogurt along with the meringue. The combination of chewy meringue and ice cream is delightful.

1 recipe	Basic Meringue (p. 70)	1 recipe
2 C	fat-free vanilla ice cream or frozen yogurt, softened	500 mL
15 oz	peach slices in juice, drained	420 g

Prepare the Basic Meringue. Trace a 12" (30 cm) circle on the inside of a clean brown paper grocery bag or a piece of parchment paper cut to fit your cookie sheet. Put the paper on an ungreased cookie sheet. Spoon the meringue into the circle. Spread so it is evenly distributed. Bake in a preheated 250°F (120°F) oven for 1 hour. Turn off the oven. Don't open the door. Leave the meringue in the oven for an additional 30 minutes. Remove to a wire rack to cool.

Carefully separate the meringue from the paper using a spatula. Put the meringue on a serving plate. Just before serving, spread the ice cream on the baked meringue and arrange peach slices in a circle at the edge. Put any remaining peach slices in the center in a pretty pattern.

Yield: 10 servings
Each serving contains:

Calories (Kcal): 83	Total fat (g): 0
Carbohydrates (g): 18	Protein (g): 3
Sodium (mg): 38	Cholesterol (mg): 2
Diabetic exchange: 1 starch/bread	

Lemon Meringue Kisses

Use a pastry bag with a ½" (13 mm) star tip for an even, professional look for kisses.

1 recipe	Basic Meringue (p. 70)	1 recipe
2 t	lemon zest, finely grated	10 mL
½ t	lemon extract	3 mL

Prepare the Basic Meringue with the following change: After peaks have formed, quickly beat in the lemon zest and extract. Cut parchment paper or brown paper grocery bags to cover the ungreased cookie sheets. Drop the meringue by teaspoonfuls (5 mL) onto the paper. Bake in a preheated 250°F (120°C) oven for 40 minutes. Turn the oven off and leave the meringues inside the closed oven for an additional 5 minutes. Remove from the oven and cool for a minute or two. Use a spatula to remove the meringues from the paper.

Yield: 5 dozen Lemon Meringue Kisses
Each kiss includes:

Calories (Kcal): 4	Total fat (g): 0
Carbohydrates (g): 0.9	Protein (g): 0
Sodium (mg): 3	Cholesterol (mg): 0
Diabetic exchange: free	

Lemon Meringue Torte

This torte has the meringue on the bottom and the top.

1 recipe	Basic Meringue (p. 70)	1 recipe
1 pkg.	sugar-free lemon pudding mix	1 pkg.
(4 servings)		(4 servings)
1¼ C	water or skim milk	1¼ C
2 t	lemon juice	10 mL

Prepare the Basic Meringue. Trace two dinner plates on parchment or the inside of a brown paper bag that has been cut the same size as your cookie sheets. Put the paper on ungreased cookie sheets. Distribute the meringue between the two circles and smooth it evenly. Bake in a preheated 250°F (120°C) oven for 1 hour. Turn off the oven but do not open the door. Leave in the oven for an additional 30 minutes. Remove to wire racks to cool.

Use a spatula to remove the torte shells from the paper. Prepare the lemon pudding according to package directions, using water or skim milk. Mix in the lemon juice. Put one of the meringues on a serving plate just before you are ready to serve. Scoop half the lemon mixture on top of the meringue. Top with the second meringue. Decorate the top with dollops of the remaining pudding mix.

Yield: 8 servings
Each serving contains:
Calories (Kcal): 33   Total fat (g): 0
Carbohydrates (g): 7   Protein (g): 2
Sodium (mg): 50   Cholesterol (mg): 0
Diabetic exchange: ½ starch/bread

Chocolate Dream Torte

A pile of meringues and fillings. Kajsa, my oldest daughter, likes it best when the meringue has been refrigerated a few hours and gets chewy.

1 recipe	Basic Meringue (p. 70)	1 recipe
1 pkg (4 servings)	sugar-free chocolate pudding mix	1 pkg. (4 servings)
1¼ C	water or skim milk	310 mL
1 C	frozen low-fat non-dairy whipped topping, thawed	250 mL

Prepare the Basic Meringue. Trace an 8" (20 cm) pie pan three times on parchment paper or the inside of a brown paper bag that has been cut the same size as your cookie sheets. Put the paper on ungreased cookie sheets. Distribute the meringue between the three circles and smooth it evenly. Bake in a preheated 250°F (120°C) oven for 40 minutes. Turn off the oven but do not open the door. Leave in the oven for an additional 30 minutes. Remove to wire racks to cool.

When you are ready to assemble the torte, remove one of the meringues carefully from the paper and place it on a serving plate. Prepare the pudding according to package directions, using the water or skim milk. (Cool, if it is a cooking recipe.) Put half the pudding on the first meringue. Smooth to the edges. Put the second meringue (with paper removed) on top and repeat with the last of the pudding and the third meringue. Cut carefully. Top each serving with a dollop of whipped topping.

Yield: 8 servings
Each serving contains:
Calories (Kcal): 74   Total fat (g): 1
Carbohydrates (g): 12   Protein (g): 4
Sodium (mg): 80   Cholesterol (mg): 1
Diabetic exchange: 1 starch/bread

Double Meringue Butterscotch Pie

There is meringue on the bottom (chunky), butterscotch in the middle (creamy and smooth), and meringue on top (chewy). What can I say except "something for everyone."

1 recipe	Basic Meringue, but use 4 egg whites (p. 70)	1 recipe
1 pkg.	sugar-free butterscotch pudding mix	1 pkg.
(4 servings)	(use the cooked variety, not the instant)	(4 servings)
2 C	skim milk	500 mL

Prepare the Basic Meringue with four egg whites and smooth two-thirds of the amount onto the inside of a 10" (25 cm) pie pan that has been coated with non-stick cooking spray. Shape the meringue into the shape of the pie pan. Save the remaining meringue in the refrigerator. Bake the pie crust in a preheated 250°F (120°C) oven for 1 hour. Turn off the oven but don't open the door; leave the pie crust in the oven to cool. Meanwhile, prepare the pudding according to package directions, using the skim milk. Just before serving, spoon the pudding into the shell. Cover with remaining uncooked meringue. Make sure the meringue topping covers the crust all the way around. Use a spoon to form peaks. Bake in a preheated 350°F (180°C) oven for 10–15 minutes. The topping will be light brown.

> Yield: 8 servings
> Each serving contains:
> Calories (Kcal): 54   Total fat (g): 0.1
> Carbohydrates (g): 10   Protein (g): 4
> Sodium (mg): 80   Cholesterol (mg): 1
> Diabetic exchange: ⅔ starch/bread

Meringue Chantilly

I sometimes put a few drops of food coloring in the whipped topping to match a party color scheme.

1 recipe	Basic Meringue (p. 70)	1 recipe
2 C	frozen low-fat non-dairy whipped topping, thawed	500 mL

Prepare the Basic Meringue. Line two ungreased cookie sheets with parchment paper or cut-up brown paper bags. Spoon the meringue onto the paper to make 12 mounds. Place the two cookie sheets into a preheated 275°F (135°C) oven. Bake for 30 minutes. Open the oven and reverse the

positions of the cookie sheets. Bake for another 30 minutes. Remove the cookie sheets from the oven. Loosen and turn each meringue over. Gently depress the center of each one with the back of a spoon. Return to the oven and bake 30 more minutes. Remove from oven and cool meringues completely. Just before serving, make sandwiches with two meringues, placing the whipped topping in between.

Yield: 6 servings
Each serving contains:

Calories (Kcal): 94	Total fat (g): 3
Carbohydrates (g): 14	Protein (g): 2
Sodium (mg): 28	Cholesterol (mg): 0

Diabetic exchange: 1 starch/bread; ½ fat

Schaum Torte

This is a great strawberry shortcake replacement.

1 recipe	Basic Meringue (p. 70)	1 recipe
1 T	sugar	15 mL
2 ¼ C	fresh strawberries or frozen whole unsweetened strawberries, sliced	310 mL
9	strawberries, hulled	9
1 C	frozen low-fat non-dairy whipped topping	250 mL

Prepare the Basic Meringue. Line ungreased cookie sheets with parchment paper or brown paper bags cut to fit cookie sheets. Drop meringue onto the paper, making 9 mounds. Use a tablespoon (15 mL) dipped in cold water to make an indentation in the top of each mound. Bake in a preheated 275°F (135°C) oven for 45 minutes. Cool thoroughly on wire racks. Meanwhile, sprinkle the sugar over the sliced strawberries, mix, and let stand. To assemble, place a meringue on a dessert plate. Scoop strawberries into the indentation. Top with a dollop of whipped topping and garnish with a whole strawberry.

Yield: 8 servings
Each serving contains:

Calories (Kcal): 72	Total fat (g): 1
Carbohydrates (g): 14	Protein (g): 2
Sodium (mg): 21	Cholesterol (mg): 0

Diabetic exchange: 1 starch/bread

Strawberry Bombe

In the same class as "Baked Alaska." Prepare this for a crowd.

1 recipe	Basic Meringue (p. 70)	1 recipe
1 quart	fat-free strawberry ice cream	950 mL
1 t	vanilla extract	5 mL

Prepare basic meringue according to the recipe. Trace a 9" (22 cm) circle on a piece of parchment paper or the inside of a brown paper bag. Cut the paper to the size of an ungreased cookie sheet. Smooth one-third of the meringue inside the circle and place the paper on the cookie sheet in a 275°F (135°C) oven for 30 minutes. Turn off the oven but do not open the door. Let the meringue sit in the oven for an additional 20 minutes. Cool on a wire rack but do not remove the paper. Just before serving time, preheat the oven to 450°F (230°C).

Heap the ice cream carefully in a mound on the meringue. Beat the vanilla extract into the remaining uncooked meringue. Smooth the uncooked meringue evenly over the strawberry ice cream dome, making sure it touches the baked meringue at all points. Bake until the meringue is a delicate brown, about 3 minutes. Serve right away, being careful to cut servings away from the brown paper.

Yield: 8 servings
Each serving contains:
Calories (Kcal): 131
Carbohydrates (g): 27
Sodium (mg): 71
Total fat (g): 0
Protein (g): 4
Cholesterol (mg): 5
Diabetic exchange: 1 starch/bread; 1 fruit

Hawaiian Alaska

There is no ice cream in this pineapple baked Alaska. An advantage is that you make individual servings.

Base
⅓ C+1 T	cold water	95 mL
¼ C+2 T	fat-free butter and oil replacement product	90 mL
2 C	flour	500 mL

Filling
3 oz	fat-free cream cheese	80 g
1 large	egg	1 large
1 t	vanilla extract	5 mL
10 slices	pineapple rings in juice, drained	10 slices

Topping
| 1 recipe | Basic Meringue (p. 70) | 1 recipe |

To prepare the base, put all the base ingredients in a mixing bowl. Mix with an electric mixer at low speed until well blended. Shape into a ball and transfer to a floured board. Roll out to ⅛" (32 mm) thickness. Cut ten 4" (10 cm) circles. Place the circles on cookie sheets that have been coated with non-stick vegetable cooking spray. Prick them all over with a fork. Bake in a preheated 450°F (230°C) oven for 8–10 minutes. Cool on a wire rack. Do not remove from cookie sheets.

Prepare the filling by blending all the filling ingredients except the pineapple rings. Place a pineapple ring on each of the bases. Spoon the filling evenly into the center of each ring. Return the cookie sheets to a preheated 400°F (200°C) oven for just 3 minutes. Quickly cover each cookie with the meringue. Return to the 400°F (200°C) oven and bake 8–10 minutes more. The meringue will be golden brown.

Yield: 10 servings
Each serving contains:
Calories (Kcal): 175
Carbohydrates (g): 36
Sodium (mg): 67
Diabetic exchange: 2 starch/bread

Total fat (g): 1
Protein (g): 5
Cholesterol (mg): 23

Ice Box Pies

Blueberry-Yogurt Pie

A substantial pie that works well after a light dinner.

1 T	unflavored gelatin	15 mL
¼ C	water	60 mL
2 large	egg yolks, slightly beaten	2 large
1 C	fat-free cottage cheese	250 mL
1 C	low-fat blueberry yogurt	250 mL
1 C	frozen low-fat non-dairy whipped topping, thawed	250 mL
4 t	aspartame sweetener	20 mL
½ C	fresh or frozen blueberries	125 mL
1	frozen pie crust, baked	1

In a small saucepan, combine the gelatin and water. Stir. Let stand for a few minutes to soften. Add the egg yolks. Cook, stirring constantly, over low heat until the mixture begins to thicken. Set aside. Put the cottage cheese into a large mixing bowl. Stir in the gelatin mixture. Add the yogurt, whipped topping, and aspartame, stirring well after each ingredient. Turn into the pie shell. Refrigerate 6–8 hours before serving. Top with fresh blueberries and additional non-dairy topping, if desired.

Yield: 8 servings
Each serving contains:
Calories (Kcal): 170   Total fat (g): 8
Carbohydrates (g): 19   Protein (g): 6
Sodium (mg): 195   Cholesterol (mg): 57
Diabetic exchange: 1 starch/bread; 1 high fat meat; 1 fat

Double Blueberry Pie

This is called double blueberry because you cook half the blueberries and not the other half. This makes for great flavor and texture.

6 oz	fat-free cream cheese	160 g
2 T	skim milk	30 mL
½ t	lemon extract	3 mL
4 C	fresh blueberries or frozen, unsweetened	1 L
1 T	lemon juice	15 mL
	water	
2 T	cornstarch	30 mL
7 t	aspartame sweetener	35 mL
1	frozen pie crust, baked	1

Put the cream cheese into a mixing bowl. Add the skim milk and lemon extract. With an electric mixer, whip until smooth and soft. Distribute the cream cheese mixture onto the bottom of the pie shell. Be careful not to damage the shell as you coat it with the cream cheese. Measure two cups (500 mL) of blueberries and put them on top of the cream cheese in the pie shell. Mash the remaining berries and put them into a two-cup (500 mL) measure. Add the teaspoon (30 mL) of lemon juice to the blueberries in the measuring cup. Add enough water so the combination of mashed blueberries, lemon juice, and water comes up to 1½ cups (375 mL). Transfer this mixture to a small saucepan. Add the cornstarch and stir to blend. Place the pan over heat and bring to a boil. Stir constantly. Cook for a minute or two until the mixture is thick. Set aside to cool. When the mixture is lukewarm, stir in the aspartame. Spoon the sauce over the fresh blueberries in the pie crust. Refrigerate for at least 3 hours. Serve with dollops of your favorite white topping, if desired.

Yield: 8 servings
Each serving contains:

Calories (Kcal): 157	Total fat (g): 5
Carbohydrates (g): 23	Protein (g): 3
Sodium (mg): 210	Cholesterol (mg): 4

Diabetic exchange: 1 starch/bread; ½ fruit; 1 fat

Apricot Cream Pie

Try decorating the top with cut pieces of dried apricots.

2 large	egg yolks, beaten lightly	2 large
1½ C	apricot nectar with no added sugar	375 mL
1 env.	unflavored gelatin	1 env.
1 T	lemon juice (fresh is best)	15 mL
2 C	frozen low-fat non-dairy whipped topping, thawed	500 mL
1	frozen pie crust, baked	1

Put the egg yolks and apricot nectar into a medium saucepan. Use a wire whisk to blend the two. Cook over medium heat, stirring constantly, until slightly thickened. Remove from heat. In a small bowl, combine the gelatin and the lemon juice. Stir and let sit for a minute or two. Add to the hot mixture. Stir. Cool for 15–20 minutes. Pour into a mixing bowl. Stir in the whipped topping. Pour into the prepared pie shell. Refrigerate 3–4 hours or until set.

Yield: 8 servings
Each serving contains:
Calories (Kcal): 165   Total fat (g): 8
Carbohydrates (g): 20   Protein (g): 2
Sodium (mg): 108   Cholesterol (mg): 53
Diabetic exchange: 1 starch/bread; ⅓ fruit; 1½ fat

Lime Chiffon Pie

The "Parrot Heads" (Jimmy Buffet fans) around my house think this is a good substitute for Key lime pie. Kristen's favorite of all.

1 pkg. (4 servings)	sugar-free lime gelatin mix	1 pkg. (4 servings)
½ C	boiling water	125 mL
1 T	lime juice (Key lime is best)	15 mL
½ C	cold water	125 mL
	ice cubes	
2 C	frozen low-fat non-dairy whipped topping, thawed	500 mL
1	frozen pie crust, baked	1

Put the gelatin powder in a large mixing bowl. Add the boiling water and stir until the powder is dissolved. Add the lime juice. Put the cold water into a one-cup measuring cup. Add ice cubes until reaching the one-cup mark. Put this water and ice mixture into a blender or food processor. Add the gelatin mixture and blend until the ice has disappeared. Add the whipped topping. Blend again until mixed. Spoon into prepared pie crust. Refrigerate at least 1 hour before serving.

Yield: 8 servings
Each serving contains:

Calories (Kcal): 124	Total fat (g): 7
Carbohydrates (g): 13	Protein (g): 1
Sodium (mg): 131	Cholesterol (mg): 0

Diabetic exchange: 1 starch/bread; 1 fat

Lemon Chiffon Pie

I think this is the best way to end a meal that features fish.

Prepare the Lime Chiffon Pie above, except use lemon gelatin mix in place of lime and lemon juice in place of Key lime juice.

Yield: 8 servings:
Each serving contains:

Calories (Kcal): 124	Total fat (g): 7
Carbohydrates (g): 13	Protein (g): 1
Sodium (mg): 131	Cholesterol (mg): 0

Diabetic exchange: 1 starch/bread; 1 fat

Raspberry Shimmer Pie

This layered pie looks and tastes spectacular. Don't be overwhelmed by the length of the directions—there is nothing tricky to do.

4 C	raspberries (fresh or frozen whole berries without syrup)	1 L
1 C	water	250 mL
3 T	cornstarch	45 mL
2 t	lemon juice	10 mL
7 t	aspartame sweetener	35 mL
3 oz	fat-free cream cheese	80 g
1 T	skim milk	15 mL
1	frozen pie crust, baked	1

Wash the fresh berries (if you are using them) very gently in cold water. Spread them to dry in a single layer on paper towels. Put 1 C (250 mL) of the raspberries and ⅔ C (165 mL) of the water into a small saucepan over medium heat. Simmer for 3–4 minutes. Strain the liquid to remove the seeds. Return the liquid to the saucepan. Add the remaining ⅓ C (80 mL) water and the cornstarch. Stir. Cook until the mixture is thick, stirring constantly. Add the lemon juice. Stir. Set aside to cool. When cool, add the aspartame and mix thoroughly.

Put the cream cheese into a mixing bowl. Add the milk. Whip until soft. Spread the cream cheese mixture very gently over the bottom of the pie crust, being careful not to damage the crust. Spread most of the reserved berries (saving a few for garnish) over the cream cheese mixture in the pie shell. Put the cooled, cooked berry mixture over the fresh berries. Refrigerate 2–3 hours. Serve with your favorite white topping, if desired. Garnish with reserved raspberries.

Yield: 8 servings
Each serving contains:

Calories (Kcal): 140	Total fat (g): 5
Carbohydrates (g): 20	Protein (g): 2
Sodium (mg): 155	Cholesterol (mg): 2

Diabetic exchange: 1 starch/bread; ½ fruit; 1 fat

Raspberry Ribbon Pie

The ribbon in the title refers to the red and white layers.

1 pkg. (4 servings)	sugar-free raspberry gelatin mix	1 pkg. (4 servings)
1¼ C	boiling water	310 mL
10 oz	frozen whole red raspberries	300 g
1 T	lemon juice	15 mL
3 oz	fat-free cream cheese	80 g
2 t	aspartame sweetener	10 mL
1 t	vanilla extract	5 mL
1 C	frozen low-fat non-dairy whipped topping, thawed	250 mL
1	frozen pie crust, baked	1

To prepare the red layers: Put the raspberry gelatin mix into a mixing bowl. Add the boiling water. Add the frozen raspberries and lemon juice. Stir until the raspberries are defrosted. Refrigerate 1–2 hours until partially set.

To prepare the white layers: In a mixing bowl, combine the cream cheese, aspartame, and vanilla. Add a spoonful of the whipped topping. Fold to mix. Continue adding the topping spoonful by spoonful, folding in each addition. Refrigerate until the white layer is partially set.

Spread half the white mixture on the bottom of the pie shell. Cover with half the red gelatin mixture. Repeat with white and red layers, ending with the white mixture. Chill until set, 3 hours or more.

> Yield: 8 servings
> Each serving contains:
> Calories (Kcal): 132　　　Total fat (g): 6
> Carbohydrates (g): 16　　Protein (g): 2
> Sodium (mg): 182　　　　Cholesterol (mg): 2
> Diabetic exchange: 1 starch/bread; 1 fat

Raspberry Cream Pie

Prepare this in the morning and let it freeze all day.

1 pkg. (4 servings)	sugar-free raspberry gelatin mix	1 pkg. (4 servings)
⅔ C	boiling water	165 mL
1½ C	sugar-free low-fat vanilla ice cream	375 mL
1½ C	frozen low-fat non-dairy whipped topping, thawed	375 mL
1 C	fresh or frozen (no sugar syrup) whole raspberries	250 mL
1	frozen pie crust, baked	1

Put the gelatin powder into a large mixing bowl. Add the boiling water. Stir until the gelatin is dissolved. Add the ice cream slowly. Stir until the mixture is smooth. Stir in the whipped topping. When well blended, add the raspberries. Transfer to the pie crust. Freeze until firm, an hour or more. For easiest cutting, run a sharp knife under hot running water between each cut. Top each slice with a dollop of whipped topping and raspberries.

Yield: 8 servings
Each serving contains:

Calories (Kcal): 140	Total fat (g): 7
Carbohydrates (g): 18	Protein (g): 1
Sodium (mg): 143	Cholesterol (mg): 0

Diabetic exchange: 1 starch/bread; 1½ fat

Hawaiian Pineapple Pie

I don't think I was ever served this in Hawaii, but the spirit of the islands is here.

20 oz	crushed pineapple in juice	570 g
1 pkg. (4 servings)	sugar-free vanilla pudding mix	1 pkg. (4 servings)
½ C	water	125 mL
1 t	butter or margarine	5 mL
1	frozen pie crust, baked	1
½ C	frozen low-fat non-dairy whipped topping	125 mL
2 T	coconut flakes (optional)	30 mL

Drain the can of pineapple pieces, saving the juice. In a saucepan, combine the pudding mix, water, and reserved pineapple juice. Cook over medium heat. Stir constantly. When mixture comes to a full boil, add the pineapple chunks and butter. Stir well. Pour into the pie crust. Cool. Just before serving, top with the non-dairy topping and sprinkle with coconut flakes, if desired.

Yield: 8 servings
Each serving contains:
Calories (Kcal): 140   Total fat (g): 6
Carbohydrates (g): 21   Protein (g): 1
Sodium (mg): 136   Cholesterol (mg): 1
Diabetic exchange: 1 starch/bread; 1 fat

Peach Cream Cheese Pie

This pie is not very sweet. It's perfect after dinner on a hot summer evening.

½ C	orange juice	125 mL
2 envs.	plain gelatin	2 envs.
2 t	orange extract	10 mL
1 C	fat-free cream cheese	250 mL
1 C	frozen low-fat non-dairy whipped topping, thawed	250 mL
16 oz	"lite" peach slices in juice, drained and chopped	450 g
1	frozen pie crust, baked	1

In a small saucepan, heat the orange juice until simmering. Pour into a blender or food processor. Add the gelatin and orange extract. Blend for 30 seconds or so before adding the cream cheese, topping, and peaches. Blend until smooth, another 20 seconds or more. Pour quickly into the pie crust. Refrigerate 3 hours or so before serving.

Yield: 8 servings
Each serving contains:
Calories (Kcal): 170   Total fat (g): 6
Carbohydrates (g): 22   Protein (g): 4
Sodium (mg): 245   Cholesterol (mg): 5
Diabetic exchange: 1 starch/bread; ½ fruit; 1 fat

Strawberry Ice Cream Pie

Let the ice cream soften before beginning the rest of the recipe.

1 pkg. (4 servings)	sugar-free strawberry gelatin powder	1 pkg. (4 servings)
⅔ C	boiling water	165 mL
2 C	sugar-free low-fat strawberry ice cream, softened	500 mL
1 C	frozen low-fat non-dairy whipped topping, thawed	250 mL
1	frozen pie crust, baked	1
1C	fresh or frozen (no sugar added) strawberries (optional)	250 mL

Put the gelatin powder into a large mixing bowl. Add the boiling water. Stir until gelatin is dissolved. Add the ice cream slowly. Stir until the mixture is smooth (except for the strawberry pieces, of course). Stir in the whipped topping by spoonfuls. Beat after each addition. A whisk works well. Spoon the mixture into the prepared pie crust. Freeze a few hours until firm. For easiest cutting, run a sharp knife under hot running water between each cut. Garnish with strawberries and whipped topping, if desired.

Yield: 8 servings
Each serving contains:

Calories (Kcal): 128	Total fat (g): 6
Carbohydrates (g): 17	Protein (g): 0.9
Sodium (mg): 148	Cholesterol (mg): 0

Diabetic exchange: 1 starch/bread; 1 fat

Banana Cream and Strawberry Pie

I find something almost sinful about bananas and strawberries together.

1 pkg. (4 servings)	sugar-free strawberry-banana gelatin mix	1 pkg. (4 servings)
⅔ C	boiling water	165 mL
2 C	sugar-free low-fat vanilla ice cream, softened	500 mL
1 C	frozen low-fat non-dairy whipped topping, thawed	250 mL
1	frozen pie crust, baked	1
1 medium	banana, sliced	1 medium
1 C	fresh strawberries, sliced	250 mL

Put the gelatin mix into a large mixing bowl. Add the boiling water and stir until the powder is dissolved. Add the ice cream slowly. Stir until smooth. Stir in the whipped topping by spoonfuls. Beat after each addition. Transfer to a prepared pie crust. Freeze until firm, at least an hour. For easiest cutting, run a sharp knife under hot running water between each cut. Just before serving, combine the banana and strawberry slices. Spoon over pie slices.

Yield: 8 servings
Each serving contains:

Calories (Kcal): 147	Total fat (g): 6
Carbohydrates (g): 22	Protein (g): 1
Sodium (mg): 148	Cholesterol (mg): 0
Diabetic exchange: 1½ fruit; 1 fat	

Strawberry Cream Cheese Pie

The cream cheese adds a smooth and rich consistency.

1 C	fat-free cream cheese	250 mL
¼ C	fruit-only strawberry jam	60 mL
½ t	almond extract, or 1 T (15 mL) almond-flavored liqueur	3 mL
1 C	frozen low-fat non-dairy whipped topping, thawed	250 mL
1	frozen pie crust, baked	1
2 C	fresh or frozen (without syrup) strawberries	500 mL

Use an electric mixer to beat together the cream cheese, jam, and almond extract or liqueur. Changing to the lowest speed, add the whipped topping. Mix until smooth. Transfer this mixture to the prepared pie crust. Smooth the top with a spoon. Cover with the strawberries. Freeze for an hour or more before serving.

Yield: 8 servings
Each serving contains:

Calories (Kcal): 156	Total fat (g): 6
Carbohydrates (g): 19	Protein (g): 3
Sodium (mg): 238	Cholesterol (mg): 5
Diabetic exchange: 1 starch/bread; 1 fat	

Strawberry Meringue Pie

A baked Alaska–style pie with strawberries. Dessert lovers will be delighted with the ice cream–meringue combination.

4 C	sugar-free, low-fat vanilla ice cream, softened	1 L
1	frozen pie crust, baked	1
3 C	fresh strawberries or frozen, unsweetened, thawed	750 mL
2 large	egg whites	2 large
¼ t	cream of tartar	2 mL
1½ t	aspartame sweetener	8 mL

Spread the ice cream into the pie shell, pushing it to the edges. Freeze all day or overnight. Just before serving, spread the strawberries on top of the ice cream and preheat the oven to 500°F (250°C). Put the egg whites, cream of tartar, and aspartame into an electric mixing bowl. Beat at high speed until the whites are stiff and form peaks but are not dry. Spoon this meringue on top of the strawberries using the spoon to make decorative peaks. Be sure all the surface is covered right up to the crust. Put the pie on a wooden bread board and place it in the oven. Bake for 5 minutes or so in the hot oven until meringue is lightly browned. Serve at once.

Yield: 8 servings
Each serving contains:

Calories (Kcal): 150	Total fat (g): 5
Carbohydrates (g): 24	Protein (g): 1
Sodium (mg): 138	Cholesterol (mg): 0

Diabetic exchange: 1 starch/bread; ½ fruit; 1 fat

Pumpkin Ice Cream Pie

If you like pumpkin you'll enjoy this frozen ice cream pie.

2 C	sugar-free low-fat vanilla ice cream, softened	500 mL
1	frozen pie crust, baked	1
5 t	aspartame sweetener	25 mL
½ t	cinnamon	3 mL
½ t	ginger	3 mL
¼ t	nutmeg	2 mL
1 C	pumpkin	250 mL

| 1 C | frozen low-fat non-dairy whipped topping, thawed | 250 mL |

Spread the softened ice cream in the bottom of the prepared pie shell, being careful not to damage the shell. Freeze. In a large mixing bowl combine the aspartame and spices. Blend in the pumpkin. Mix well. Add the non-dairy whipped topping. Fold until well mixed. Spread this mixture over the ice cream. Freeze 2–3 hours. Put out at room temperature for a half hour before cutting.

Yield: 8 servings
Each serving contains:

Calories (Kcal): 136	Total fat (g): 6
Carbohydrates (g): 18	Protein (g): 0.9
Sodium (mg): 120	Cholesterol (mg): 0
Diabetic exchange: 1 fruit; 1½ fat	

Frozen Pumpkin Pie

My mom liked this for Thanksgiving. She thought it was nice to have something cold and refreshing after a heavy meal.

2 C	no-sugar low-fat vanilla ice cream or frozen yogurt, thawed	500 mL
2 C	frozen low-fat non-dairy whipped topping, thawed	500 mL
1 C	canned pumpkin	250 mL
2 t	aspartame sweetener	10 mL
1 t	cinnamon	5 mL
½ t	ginger	3 mL
½ t	cloves	3 mL
1	frozen pie crust, baked	1

Put the ice cream, topping, pumpkin, aspartame, and spices into a mixing bowl. Mix at medium speed until well blended. Pour into a pie shell. Freeze 3 hours or more, until firm.

Yield: 8 servings
Each serving contains:

Calories (Kcal): 153	Total fat (g): 7
Carbohydrates (g): 20	Protein (g): 0.9
Sodium (mg): 120	Cholesterol (mg): 0
Diabetic exchange: 1 starch/bread; ½ fruit; 1 fat	

Butterscotch Pie

Although this pie has pumpkin, the flavor of butterscotch is dominant and delicious.

1 T	unflavored gelatin	5 mL
1½ C	skim milk	325 mL
3 oz	fat-free cream cheese	80 g
1½ C	canned pumpkin pie filling	325 mL
2 large	eggs or equivalent egg substitute	2 large
1 pkg. (4 servings)	sugar-free butterscotch pudding mix (not instant)	1 pkg. (4 servings)
2 C	frozen low-fat non-dairy whipped topping, thawed	500 mL
1	frozen pie crust, baked	1

Put the gelatin in a small mixing bowl. Add ½ C (125 mL) milk and stir. Set aside while the gelatin softens. In the bowl of an electric mixer, combine the cream cheese, pumpkin, and eggs. Beat until smooth. In a heavy-bottomed saucepan, combine the remaining 1 cup (250 mL) of milk and the pudding mix. Add the pumpkin filling and the gelatin. Cook over medium heat until the mixture bubbles and thickens. Put the pan in the refrigerator to cool but do not allow it to set, 45 minutes or so. Fold in the whipped topping. Spoon into a prepared pie crust. Chill overnight or for several hours.

> Yield: 8 servings
> Each serving contains:
> Calories (Kcal): 179   Total fat (g): 8
> Carbohydrates (g): 17   Protein (g): 5
> Sodium (mg): 221   Cholesterol (mg): 56
> Diabetic exchange: 1 high-fat meat; 1 fruit

Chocolate Chocolate Pie

I used Hershey's low-sugar, no-fat chocolate syrup in this recipe. It worked very nicely.

1½ C	cold skim milk	375 mL
2 pkgs.	sugar-free chocolate pudding mix	2 pkgs.
(4-serving size)		(4-serving size)
1¼ C	water or skim milk	310 mL
1	frozen pie crust, baked	1
½ C	fat-free cream cheese	125 mL
1 T	cold skim milk	15 mL
2 T	low-sugar no-fat chocolate syrup	30 mL
1½ C	frozen low-fat non-dairy whipped topping	375 mL

Combine milk and pudding mixes in a mixing bowl. Beat with an electric mixer on medium speed until very thick. Turn into pie crust. Put the cream cheese and tablespoon of milk into the mixing bowl. Beat on high speed until the mixture is smooth. Using the lowest speed, mix in the syrup and whipped topping. Pour this mixture on top of the pudding mixture in the pie crust. Refrigerate 3 hours or more.

Yield: 8 servings
Each serving contains:
Calories (Kcal): 151   Total fat (g): 7
Carbohydrates (g): 18   Protein (g): 4
Sodium (mg): 254   Cholesterol (mg): 4
Diabetic exchange: 1 starch/bread; 1 fat

Coffee-and-Cream Pie

If coffee in a cup tasted this good, I'd drink a lot more of it. This pie tastes the way I always imagine coffee in a cup is going to taste. To cut the fat down to practically nothing, try fat-free whipped topping.

3 C	frozen low-fat non-dairy whipped topping, thawed	750 mL
2 T	instant coffee powder	30 mL
1 t	vanilla	5 mL
¼ C	cold water	60 mL
1 env.	unflavored gelatin	1 env.
1	frozen pie crust, baked	1
½ C	toasted coconut flakes (optional)	125 mL

Put the topping, coffee powder, and vanilla into a mixing bowl. Beat until blended. Put the cold water into a small saucepan. Sprinkle the gelatin onto the water. Let stand a minute or two. Put the saucepan over a low heat and stir until the gelatin is thoroughly dissolved. Pour the gelatin into the coffee mixture and beat again, until the gelatin is blended in. Pour the mixture into the pie crust. Sprinkle the coconut over the top, if desired. Refrigerate 1 hour or more before serving.

Yield: 8 servings
Each serving contains:
Calories (Kcal): 160   Total fat (g): 9
Carbohydrates (g): 15   Protein (g): 1
Sodium (mg): 106   Cholesterol (mg): 0
Diabetic exchange: 1 starch/bread; 2 fat

Cocoa Chiffon Pie

This needs at least eight hours to chill. Prepare it the night before you plan to serve it or in the morning if you want to serve it it in the evening. It's worth planning ahead.

1 env.	unflavored gelatin	1 env.
3 T	unsweetened cocoa powder	45 mL
1¾ C	skim milk	435 mL
1 t	vanilla extract	5 mL
1½ C	frozen low-fat non-dairy whipped topping, thawed	375 mL
1½ t	aspartame sweetener	8 mL
1	frozen pie crust, baked	1

In a medium saucepan, mix together the gelatin, cocoa powder, and skim milk. Let stand for 5 minutes or so. Place over low heat. Stir with a wire whisk until the gelatin is dissolved, about 5 minutes. Remove from heat and stir in the vanilla. Refrigerate the mixture while preparing the rest of the pie. Put the whipped topping and aspartame in a mixing bowl. Mix to combine. Add the cocoa mixture. Mix at the lowest speed until blended. Turn into prepared pie crust. Refrigerate 8 hours or overnight before serving.

Yield: 8 servings
Each serving contains:
Calories (Kcal): 145   Total fat (g): 7
Carbohydrates (g): 16   Protein (g): 3
Sodium (mg): 133   Cholesterol (mg): 1
Diabetic exchange: 1 starch/bread; 1½ fat

Gelatin

Raspberry Cream Gelatin

The sour cream makes this very mousse-like. Save a few raspberries to garnish with mint leaves for a "company" look.

1 pkg. (4 servings)	sugar-free raspberry gelatin mix	1 pkg. (4 servings)
1 C	boiling water	250 mL
½ C	fat-free sour cream	125 mL
½ C	cold water	125 mL
½ C	frozen raspberries, thawed	125 mL

Put the gelatin powder in a large mixing bowl. Add the boiling water and stir until the powder is dissolved. Add the sour cream and cold water. Stir to mix. Arrange the raspberries in four dessert bowls. Pour the gelatin mixture over the raspberries. Chill until set, about 3–4 hours.

> Yield: 4 servings
> Each serving contains:
> Calories (Kcal): 31   Total fat (g): 0.1
> Carbohydrates (g): 7   Protein (g): 2
> Sodium (mg): 83   Cholesterol (mg): 0
> Diabetic exchange: ½ starch/bread

Strawberry Yogurt Dessert

The yogurt adds a creamy texture.

1 pkg. (4 servings)	sugar-free strawberry gelatin mix	1 pkg. (4 servings)
¾ C	boiling water	185 mL
½ C	cold water	125 mL
	ice cubes	
1 C	fat-free yogurt, plain or vanilla	250 mL
½ C	fresh strawberries, hulled and sliced	125 mL
4	mint leaves (optional)	4

Put the gelatin powder into a large mixing bowl. Add the boiling water and stir until the gelatin is dissolved. Put the cold water into a two-cup (500 mL) measure. Add enough ice cubes until the measuring cup is 1¼ cups (310 mL) full. Put the cold water and ice into a food processor. Add the gelatin mixture. Blend until the ice cubes almost disappear. Add the yogurt and blend again. Distribute the strawberry slices on four dessert dishes. Pour the yogurt and gelatin mixture over the fruit. Chill for 1–2 hours. Top with your favorite white topping and garnish with mint leaves and strawberry slices, if desired.

Yield: 4 servings
Each serving contains:

Calories (Kcal): 40	Total fat (g): 0.1
Carbohydrates (g): 8	Protein (g): 0.6
Sodium (mg): 100	Cholesterol (mg): 2
Diabetic exchange: ½ fruit	

Ginger-Strawberry Cooler

Ginger is a flavor favored by people who live in tropical climates because it's cooling. Try making this easy dessert or snack for the hottest days.

1 pkg.	sugar-free strawberry-kiwi gelatin mix	1 pkg.
(4 servings)		(4 servings)
1 C	boiling water	250 mL
¼ t	ground ginger	2 mL
1 C	sugar-free ginger ale	250 mL
½ C	fresh strawberries or frozen no-sugar-added, thawed and then sliced	125 mL

Put the gelatin powder into a large mixing bowl. Add the boiling water and ginger. Stir until the gelatin is dissolved. Add the ginger ale and mix. Arrange the strawberries in four dessert bowls. Pour the gelatin mixture over the strawberries. Chill for 3–4 hours. Top with your favorite white topping, if desired.

Yield: 4 servings
Each serving contains:

Calories (Kcal): 10	Total fat (g): 0.1
Carbohydrates (g): 3	Protein (g): 0.6
Sodium (mg): 57	Cholesterol (mg): 0
Diabetic exchange: free	

Strawberry Layered Dessert

Although this recipe calls for sugar-free, fat-free ice cream, you can use sugar-free, fat-free frozen yogurt instead.

1 pkg. (4 servings)	sugar-free strawberry-banana gelatin mix	1 pkg. (4 servings)
¾ C	boiling water	185 mL
½ C	cold water	125 mL
	ice cubes	
½ C	sugar-free low-fat vanilla ice cream	125 mL
½ C	fresh strawberries, hulled and sliced	125 mL

Put the gelatin powder into a large mixing bowl. Add the boiling water and stir until dissolved. Put the cold water into a two-cup (500 mL) measure. Add enough ice cubes until the measuring cup is 1¼ cups (310 mL) full. Put the cold water and ice into a food processor. Add the gelatin mixture. Blend until the ice cubes almost disappear. Divide this gelatin mixture in half. Add the ice cream to one half and the strawberries to the other. Mix until smooth. In each of four individual dessert dishes, spoon a layer of fruit mixture. Spoon a creamy layer on top. Chill until set. This will take an hour or so. Top with your favorite white topping.

> Yield: 4 servings
> Each serving contains:
> Calories (Kcal): 22   Total fat (g): 0.1
> Carbohydrates (g): 6   Protein (g): 0.6
> Sodium (mg): 66   Cholesterol (mg): 0
> Diabetic exchange: ½ fruit

Strawberry-Banana Cubes

Kids love these. For special effects use cookie cutters.

1 pkg. (4 servings)	sugar-free strawberry-banana gelatin mix	1 pkg. (4 servings)
¾ C	boiling water	185 mL
¾ C	cold water	185 mL
1 medium	banana, sliced	1 medium
½ C	fresh strawberries, sliced (optional)	125 mL

Put the strawberry-banana gelatin powder into a large mixing bowl. Add the boiling water and stir until the powder is dissolved. Add the cold water and stir. Arrange the fruit in an 8×8 inch (20×20 cm) brownie pan. Pour the gelatin over the fruit. Chill for 3–4 hours until the mixture sets. Cut into cubes and arrange the cubes in a circle around the edge of the plate. Optional: Place fresh fruit or a dash of your favorite white topping in the center.

Yield: 4 servings
Each serving contains:

Calories (Kcal): 36	Total fat (g): 0.2
Carbohydrates (g): 10	Protein (g): 0.9
Sodium (mg): 58	Cholesterol (mg): 0
Diabetic exchange: ½ fruit	

Pear and Banana Gelatin Dessert

If you like your fruit floating in gelatin, let it begin to set for 20–30 minutes and then stir in the fruit and nuts. No one in my house minds the fruit at the bottom.

1 pkg.	sugar-free strawberry-banana gelatin mix	1 pkg.
(4 servings)		(4 servings)
1 C	boiling water	250 mL
½ t	rum-flavored extract	3 mL
1 C	cold water	250 mL
½ C	fresh pears, sliced, or canned "lite" pears, drained	125 mL
½ C	bananas, sliced	125 mL
2 T	walnuts, chopped fine chopped (optional)	30 mL

Put the gelatin powder into a large mixing bowl. Add the boiling water and rum extract. Stir until the gelatin is dissolved. Add the cold water and mix. Arrange the fruit and the nuts (if used) in four individual dessert bowls. Pour the gelatin mixture over the fruit. Chill until firm, about 3–4 hours. Top with your favorite white topping, if desired.

Yield: 4 servings
Each serving contains:

Calories (Kcal): 43	Total fat (g): 0.2
Carbohydrates (g): 12	Protein (g): 0.9
Sodium (mg): 59	Cholesterol (mg): 0
Diabetic exchange: ⅔ fruit	

Lime and Banana Gelatin Dessert

If you want the bananas to "float," wait to add them after the gelatin has started to jell.

1 pkg. (4 servings)	sugar-free lime gelatin mix	1 pkg. (4 servings)
1 C	boiling water	250 mL
½ C	cold water	125 mL
½ C	fat-free sour cream	125 mL
1 medium	banana, sliced	1 medium

Put the gelatin powder into a large mixing bowl. Add the boiling water and stir until the powder is dissolved. Add the cold water and the sour cream and stir until the sour cream is completely blended. Arrange the banana slices in four dessert dishes. Pour the gelatin mixture over the bananas. Chill for 3–4 hours.

> Yield: 4 servings
> Each serving contains:
> Calories (Kcal): 50   Total fat (g): 0.1
> Carbohydrates (g): 12   Protein (g): 2
> Sodium (mg): 83   Cholesterol (mg): 0
> Diabetic exchange: ½ starch/bread

Key Lime Pudding

Light and tart, this pudding is refreshing.

1 pkg. (4 servings)	sugar-free lime gelatin mix	1 pkg. (4 servings)
¾ C	boiling water	185 mL
1 T	lime juice (Key lime juice is great)	15 mL
½ C	cold water	125 mL
	ice cubes	
1¾ C	frozen low-fat non-dairy whipped topping	440 mL

Put the gelatin powder into a large mixing bowl. Add the boiling water and stir until the powder is dissolved. Add the lime juice. Put the cold water into a two-cup (500 mL) measuring cup. Add ice cubes until the measure is 1¼ cups (310 mL) full. Put the water and ice mixture into a blender or food processor. Add the gelatin mixture and blend until the ice has almost disappeared. Add non-dairy topping. Blend again until mixed. Pour into 8 serving dishes. Chill until set, about 1 hour.

Yield: 8 servings
Each serving contains:

Calories (Kcal): 37	Total fat (g): 2
Carbohydrates (g): 5	Protein (g): 0.3
Sodium (mg): 29	Cholesterol (mg): 0
Diabetic exchange: ½ fat	

Lemon Pudding

A nice variation of lime pudding. For a big crowd I make one recipe of each.

Prepare Key Lime Pudding, but use sugar-free lemon gelatin mix in place of the lime gelatin mix and use lemon juice in place of the Key lime juice.

Yield: 8 servings
Each serving contains:

Calories (Kcal): 37	Total fat (g): 2
Carbohydrates (g): 5	Protein (g): 0.3
Sodium (mg): 29	Cholesterol (mg): 0
Diabetic exchange: ½ fat	

Café-au-Lait Squares

This recipe is adapted from one of my grandmother's. I've tried it with fla-vored coffees, such as vanilla and hazelnut, and it's terrific. I sometimes pre-pare these in my best coffee cups instead of a square pan. Chill as usual.

4 envs.	unflavored gelatin	4 envs.
1 C	skim milk	250 mL
1½ C	strong coffee	375 mL
6 T	semisweet chocolate chips (use low-fat chips, if available)	90 mL
6 pkgs.	saccharin or acesulfame-K sugar substitute	6 pkgs.
1½ t	vanilla extract	8 mL

Put the unflavored gelatin into a medium mixing bowl. Add the skim milk. Stir and set aside. In a small saucepan, bring the coffee to a boil. Pour over the gelatin. Stir until the gelatin is completely dissolved. Add the other ingredients. Coat an 8" (20 cm) square baking pan with non-stick vegetable spray. Pour the batter into the pan. Chill until firm. Cut into 9 squares.

> Yield: 9 squares
> Each square contains:
> Calories (Kcal): 81   Total fat (g): 3
> Carbohydrates (g): 9   Protein (g): 4
> Sodium (mg): 27   Cholesterol (mg): 0
> Diabetic exchange: ½ high fat meat; ½ fruit

Easy Mixed Fruit–Gelatin Dessert

The name says it all.

1 pkg. (4 servings)	sugar-free orange gelatin mix	1 pkg. (4 servings)
1 C	boiling water	250 mL
1 C	cold water	250 mL
½ C	canned "lite" fruit chunks, drained	125 mL

Put the orange gelatin powder into a large mixing bowl. Stir in the boiling water and mix until the powder is dissolved. Add the cold water and mix. Arrange the fruit in four dessert dishes. Pour the gelatin mixture over the fruit. Chill for 3–4 hours. Top with a garnish of your favorite white topping, if desired.

Yield: 4 servings
Each serving contains:

Calories (Kcal): 15	Total fat (g): 0
Carbohydrates (g): 5	Protein (g): 0.7
Sodium (mg): 59	Cholesterol (mg): 0
Diabetic exchange: free	

Orange Cottage Cheese Dessert

Not too sweet. My mother loves this dessert.

1 pkg. (4 servings)	sugar-free orange gelatin mix	1 pkg. (4 servings)
1 C	boiling water	250 mL
1 C	cold water	125 mL
1 C	fat-free small curd cottage cheese	125 mL
2 C	orange sections, diced	500 mL

Put the gelatin powder into a large mixing bowl. Add the boiling water. Stir until the gelatin dissolves. Add the cold water. Stir. Place the gelatin mixture into a food processor or blender. Add the cottage cheese. Blend until the mixture is smooth. Pour into four dessert dishes. Chill 3–4 hours. Garnish with the diced orange sections just before serving.

Yield: 4 servings
Each serving contains:

Calories (Kcal): 79	Total fat (g): 0.1
Carbohydrates (g): 16	Protein (g): 8
Sodium (mg): 209	Cholesterol (mg): 5
Diabetic exchange: 1 milk	

Creamy Melon Gelatin Dessert

I make this when I have a leftover melon or cantaloupe.

1 pkg. (4 servings)	sugar-free lime gelatin mix	1 pkg. (4 servings)
1 C	boiling water	250 mL
½ C	sugar-free low-fat vanilla ice cream	125 mL
½ C	cold water	125 mL
½ C	cantaloupe or honeydew melon pieces, fresh or frozen	125 mL

Put the gelatin powder into a large mixing bowl. Add the boiling water and stir until the gelatin is dissolved. Add the ice cream and cold water. Stir to mix. Arrange the pieces of melon in four dessert dishes. Pour the gelatin mixture over the fruit. Chill 3–4 hours.

> Yield: 4 servings
> Each serving contains:
> Calories (Kcal): 23   Total fat (g): 0.1
> Carbohydrates (g): 7   Protein (g): 0.7
> Sodium (mg): 68   Cholesterol (mg): 0
> Diabetic exchange: ½ fruit

Piña Colada Squares

There is something about the piña colada taste and texture that's so tropical. You can pour into dessert or wineglasses (instead of the square pan) before chilling, as an alternative.

4 envs.	unflavored gelatin	4 envs.
6 pkgs.	saccharin or acesulfame-K sugar substitute	6 pkgs.
2½ C	unsweetened pineapple juice	625 mL
1 C	frozen low-fat non-dairy whipped topping	250 mL
1 t	coconut extract	5 mL
½ t	rum extract	3 mL

Put the unflavored gelatin and the sugar substitute into a mixing bowl. Add ½ C (125 mL) pineapple juice. Stir. Set aside. Meanwhile, in a small saucepan bring the pineapple juice to a boil. Add the pineapple mixture all at once to the gelatin mixture, stirring to combine. Stir in the whipped top-

ping and extracts. Coat an 8" (20 cm) square pan with non-stick vegetable cooking spray. Pour the batter into the pan. Chill until firm. Cut into 9 squares.

Yield: 9 squares
Each square contains:
Calories (Kcal): 99   Total fat (g): 2
Carbohydrates (g): 18   Protein (g): 3
Sodium (mg): 18   Cholesterol (mg): 0
Diabetic exchange: 1 starch/bread; ½ fat

"Creamsicle" Gelatin

Do you love creamsicles? This recipe will get you close in taste for very few calories!

1 pkg. (4 servings)	sugar-free orange gelatin mix	1 pkg. (4 servings)
1 C	boiling water	250 mL
½ C	vanilla sugar-free low-fat ice cream	125 mL
½ C	cold water	125 mL
¼ C	orange sections	60 mL

Put the gelatin powder into a large mixing bowl. Add the boiling water and stir until the powder is dissolved. Add the ice cream and cold water. Stir to mix. Pour into four dessert bowls. Chill until firm, 3–4 hours. Garnish with orange sections.

Yield: 4 servings
Each serving contains:
Calories (Kcal): 22   Total fat (g): 0
Carbohydrates (g): 6   Protein (g): 0.6
Sodium (mg): 66   Cholesterol (mg): 0
Diabetic exchange: ½ fruit

Cream Puffs

Cream Puff Pastry

You won't believe how easy cream puffs are until you prepare them yourself. This recipe is practically foolproof and needs no exotic kitchen equipment.

1 C	water	250 mL
⅓ C	canola oil	80 mL
1 C	flour	250 mL
4 large	eggs or equivalent egg substitute	4 large
1 t	butter extract	5 mL
1 t	vanilla extract	5 mL

Put the water and canola oil in a medium saucepan. Heat to a rolling boil. Lower the heat and add the flour all at once, stirring with a wooden spoon until the mixture forms a ball. Remove from the heat. With an electric mixer, beat in the eggs one at a time. Add the extracts. Using a spoon, drop 12 cream puffs onto an ungreased cookie sheet. Bake in a 400°F (200°C) oven for 10 minutes. Reduce the heat to 350°F (180°C) and bake for 25 minutes longer. Turn off the oven but do not remove cream puffs until they are quite firm to the touch. Cool them away from drafts. To fill, cut the puffs horizontally, using a sharp knife. If any damp dough remains inside, scoop it out before filling.

Yield: 12 Cream Puffs
Each puff contains:
Calories (Kcal): 117   Total fat (g): 8
Carbohydrates (g): 8   Protein (g): 3
Sodium (mg): 22   Cholesterol (mg): 71
Diabetic exchange: ½ starch/bread; ¼ high fat meat; 1 fat

Light Chocolate Cream Puffs

Very impressive, and easier than pie!

1 recipe	Cream Puff Pastry (p. 110)	1 recipe
1 recipe	Chocolate Mousse Pudding (p. 52)	1 recipe
1 recipe	Chocolate Glaze (p. 35)	1 recipe
	or Napoleon Fudge Topping recipe (p. 37)	

Prepare the cream puffs from the puff pastry, make the Chocolate Mousse Pudding, and the glaze or fudge topping. Assemble the cream puffs by putting the pudding inside the pastry and drizzling the glaze or fudge topping over the top.

Yield: 12 Light Chocolate Cream Puffs
    Each puff contains:
    Calories (Kcal): 139   Total fat (g): 15
    Carbohydrates (g): 11   Protein (g): 4
    Sodium (mg): 62   Cholesterol (mg): 71
    Diabetic exchange: 2 vegetable; 3 fat

Light Mocha Cream Puffs

For those who love that mocha flavor.

1 recipe	Cream Puff Pastry (p. 110)	1 recipe
1 recipe	Mocha Tart Filling (p. 32)	1 recipe
1 recipe	Chocolate Glaze (p. 35)	1 recipe
	or Napoleon Fudge Topping (p. 37)	

Prepare the cream puff pastry and the mocha filling. Bake the cream puffs. Assemble by putting the filling inside the cream puffs. Drizzle chocolate glaze or fudge topping over the top of the cream puffs.

Yield: 12 Light Mocha Cream Puffs
    Each puff contains:
    Calories (Kcal): 125   Total fat (g): 8
    Carbohydrates (g): 10   Protein (g): 4
    Sodium (mg): 40   Cholesterol (mg): 71
    Diabetic exchange: 2 vegetable; 1½ fat

Traditional Cream Puffs

These look and taste like the cream puffs sold in bakeries.

1 recipe	Cream Puff Pastry (p. 110)	1 recipe
1 recipe	Vanilla Tart Filling (p. 45)	1 recipe
1 recipe	Chocolate Glaze (p. 35)	
	or Napoleon Fudge Topping (p. 37)	1 recipe

Prepare the puff pastry, tart filling, and one of the toppings. Bake the cream puffs. Assemble by putting tart filling inside the puffs, covering with the tops, and drizzling with Chocolate Glaze or Napoleon Fudge.

Yield: 12 Traditional Cream Puffs
Each puff contains:

Calories (Kcal): 176	Total fat (g): 10
Carbohydrates (g): 15	Protein (g): 5
Sodium (mg): 78	Cholesterol (mg): 94

Diabetic exchange: 1 starch/bread; 2 fat

Mocha Cream Puffs

A more pronounced coffee flavor.

1 recipe	Cream Puff Pastry (p. 110)	1 recipe
1 recipe	Mocha Tart Filling (p. 32)	1 recipe
1 recipe	Mocha Glaze (p. 33)	1 recipe

Prepare the puff pastry, Mocha Tart Filling, and Mocha Glaze. Bake the cream puffs. Assemble by putting the coffee filling inside the puffs, covering with the tops, and drizzling with glaze.

Yield: 12 Mocha Cream Puffs
Each puff contains:

Calories (Kcal): 125	Total fat (g): 8
Carbohydrates (g): 10	Protein (g): 4
Sodium (mg): 39	Cholesterol (mg): 71

Diabetic exchange: 2 vegetable; 1½ fat

Strawberry Cream Puffs

An easy alternative to strawberry shortcake and very pretty.

1 recipe	Cream Puff Pastry (p. 110)	1 recipe
3 C	fresh strawberries, or frozen whole strawberries without sugar	750 mL
1 C	frozen low-fat non-dairy whipped topping	250 mL

Make and bake the cream puffs. Put ¼ C (60 mL) strawberries in each puff. Put the top back on. Add a dollop of whipped topping to the top.

Yield: 12 Strawberry Cream Puffs
Each puff contains:
Calories (Kcal): 142   Total fat (g): 7
Carbohydrates (g): 12   Protein (g): 3
Sodium (mg): 22   Cholesterol (mg): 71
Diabetic exchange: 1 starch/bread; 1½ fat

Banana Cream Puffs

If you have bananas, all the rest of the ingredients are "on the shelf." I love this for unexpected guests.

1 recipe	Cream Puff Pastry (p. 110)	1 recipe
1 recipe	Vanilla Tart Filling (p. 45)	1 recipe
4 medium	bananas, peeled and sliced	4 medium
3 t	lemon juice	15 mL
1 C	frozen low-fat non-dairy whipped topping	250 mL

Prepare the cream puffs and Vanilla Tart Filling. Bake the cream puffs. Put the banana slices into a medium mixing bowl. Pour the lemon juice over the bananas and toss to distribute the lemon juice evenly. Add the pudding and mix. Spoon this pudding mixture into the cream puffs. Put the cream puff tops on and add a dollop of white topping.

Yield: 12 Banana Cream Puffs
Each puff contains:
Calories (Kcal): 216   Total fat (g): 10
Carbohydrates (g): 24   Protein (g): 5
Sodium (mg): 66   Cholesterol (mg): 94
Diabetic exchange: 1½ starch/bread; 2 fat

Cream Puffs with Raspberry Sauce

The raspberry sauce is striking against the light colors of the puffs and filling and adds a contrasting flavor and texture, too.

1 recipe	Cream Puff Pastry (p. 110)	1 recipe
1 recipe	Vanilla Tart Filling (p. 45)	1 recipe
1 recipe	Raspberry Sauce (p. 75)	1 recipe

Prepare the cream puffs, tart filling, and Raspberry Sauce. Bake the cream puffs. Fill them with the filling and put the tops back on. Spoon the sauce over the puffs.

Yield: 12 Cream Puffs with Raspberry Sauce
Each puff contains:
Calories (Kcal): 199   Total fat (g): 10
Carbohydrates (g): 20   Protein (g): 5
Sodium (mg): 71   Cholesterol (mg): 94
Diabetic exchange: 1 starch/bread; 1 vegetable; 2 fat

New Zealand Cream Puffs

Kiwis are ready to eat when they yield to gentle pressure. Eat them at their sweetest.

1 recipe	Cream Puff Pastry (p. 110)	1 recipe
4	kiwi fruit, peeled and chopped	4
2 C	fresh strawberries, hulled and sliced	500 mL
2 C	frozen low-fat non-dairy whipped topping, thawed	500 mL

Prepare the cream puffs according to the directions. When ready to assemble, put the chopped kiwis and sliced strawberries in a bowl. Add the whipped topping and fold the mixture together. Spoon the fruit mixture into the cream puffs. Put the tops back on and serve immediately.

Yield: 12 New Zealand Cream Puffs
Each puff contains:
Calories (Kcal): 167   Total fat (g): 9
Carbohydrates (g): 16   Protein (g): 4
Sodium (mg): 23   Cholesterol (mg): 71
Diabetic exchange: 1 starch/bread; 2 fat

Icy Peach Cream Puffs

Only the puffs are prepared ahead of time for this. Prepare them in the morning and refrigerate the peaches. Assemble everything after serving dinner.

1 recipe	Cream Puff Pastry (p. 110)	1 recipe
3 C	sugar-free low-fat vanilla ice cream or frozen yogurt	750 mL
30 oz	canned peaches packed in juice, drained, chopped and chilled	850 g

Prepare the basic cream puff recipe. Bake the puffs. When ready to serve, put ¼ C (60 mL) ice cream in each puff. Distribute the chopped peaches over the ice cream. Put on the tops and serve immediately.

Yield: 12 Icy Peach Cream Puffs
Each puff contains:
Calories (Kcal): 172 — Total fat (g): 8
Carbohydrates (g): 22 — Protein (g): 4
Sodium (mg): 39 — Cholesterol (mg): 71
Diabetic exchange: 1½ starch/bread; 1 fat

Frozen Chocolate Cream Puffs

Prepare these ahead of time and freeze them. I move them to the refrigerator just as I'm putting dinner on the table. They are perfect for dessert.

1 recipe	Cream Puff Pastry (p. 110)	1 recipe
3 C	cold skim milk	750 mL
2 pkgs. (4-serving size)	sugar-free chocolate pudding mix	2 pkgs. (4-serving size)

Prepare the basic cream puffs. Bake them. In a medium mixing bowl, beat together the skim milk and the pudding mix with an electric mixer until thick. Scoop the pudding into the cream puffs. Put the tops on and freeze. When frozen, put them in plastic bags until you are ready to use them.

Yield: 12 Frozen Chocolate Cream Puffs
Each puff contains:
Calories (Kcal): 141 — Total fat (g): 8
Carbohydrates (g): 12 — Protein (g): 6
Sodium (mg): 90 — Cholesterol (mg): 72
Diabetic exchange: 1 milk; 1½ fat

Frozen Raspberry Cream Puffs

These make-ahead cream puffs are perfect to freeze and eat one at a time.

1 recipe	Cream Puff Pastry (p. 110)	1 recipe	
1 recipe	Raspberry Filling for Raspberry Cream Pie (p. 90)	1 recipe	

Prepare the basic cream puffs and the filling for the raspberry cream pie. Bake the puffs. Spoon the filling into the cream puffs, put on the tops, and freeze them. After they are frozen, put them in plastic freezer bags. Remove from the freezer at the beginning of dinner and they will be ready by dessert time.

Yield: 12 Frozen Raspberry Cream Puffs
Each puff contains:
Calories (Kcal): 156   Total fat (g): 9
Carbohydrates (g): 15   Protein (g): 3
Sodium (mg): 49   Cholesterol (mg): 71
Diabetic exchange: 1 starch/bread; 2 fat

Frozen Strawberry Cream Puffs

Remove as many as you need from the freezer when you get dinner ready. I make these on rainy Sunday afternoons and use them for rushed after-work dinners.

1 recipe	Cream Puff Pastry (p. 110)	1 recipe	
1 recipe	Strawberry Ice Cream Pie Filling (p. 92)	1 recipe	

Prepare the basic cream puffs and the strawberry ice cream pie filling from the Strawberry Ice Cream Pie recipe. Spoon the filling inside the baked cream puffs. Put the tops on and freeze. After freezing the puffs, put them in plastic freezer bags.

Yield: 12 Frozen Strawberry Cream Puffs
Each puff contains:
Calories (Kcal): 148   Total fat (g): 8
Carbohydrates (g): 14   Protein (g): 3
Sodium (mg): 52   Cholesterol (mg): 71
Diabetic exchange: 1 starch/bread; 1½ fat

Dressed-Up Angels

Snowball Cake

Impressive! Prepare this any time you want to show off. It looks fabulous on a buffet table.

1 pkg.	sugar-free strawberry gelatin mix	1 pkg.
(4 servings)		(4 servings)
1 C	hot water	250 mL
1 C	cold water	250 mL
1 C	frozen low-fat non-dairy whipped topping, thawed	250 mL
2 C	fresh strawberries or frozen, sugar-free, defrosted	500 mL
1	angel food cake, cut into 1" (2.5 cm) cubes	1

Prepare the gelatin by putting the powder into a mixing bowl. Add the hot water and stir until the powder is dissolved. Add the cold water and stir to combine. Refrigerate an hour or so until partially set. In another bowl, fold together the whipped topping and the strawberries. Fold into the partially set gelatin. Return to the refrigerator.

Line a deep mixing bowl with long pieces of waxed paper. The pieces should extend over the edge, travel down the inside of the bowl and up the other side, extending past the rims. Use several overlapping strips so the inside of the bowl is totally covered. Alternate layers of the gelatin mixture with cake cubes in the bowl. Refrigerate 8 hours or overnight. Before serving, put a cake plate upside down on top of the bowl. Turn the whole thing over. Peel off the waxed paper carefully.

Yield: 16 servings
Each serving contains:

Calories (Kcal): 112	Total fat (g): 0.7
Carbohydrates (g): 25	Protein (g): 3
Sodium (mg): 204	Cholesterol (mg): 0

Diabetic exchange: 1 starch/bread; ½ fruit

Gourmet Strawberries and Mint

Not your run-of-the-mill strawberry shortcake. This is a nice treat at a luncheon.

4 C	fresh strawberries, sliced	1 L
2 T	powdered sugar	30 mL
1 T	fresh mint leaves, finely chopped	15 mL
1 C	fat-free sugar-free lemon yogurt	250 mL
¼ C	fat-free sour cream	60 mL
1	angel food cake, cut in 16 slices	1

Mix the strawberries, powdered sugar, and mint together in a mixing bowl. Set aside for an hour at room temperature. This will cause the strawberries to let out their juice. When you are ready to serve, mix the yogurt and sour cream together in a small bowl. Put one slice of cake on each of 8 dessert plates. Put a spoonful of strawberries on top and then the second slice of cake. Top with the rest of the strawberries and distribute the yogurt–sour cream mixture.

Yield: 8 servings
Each serving contains:
Calories (Kcal): 161   Total fat (g): 0.3
Carbohydrates (g): 36   Protein (g): 3
Sodium (mg): 272   Cholesterol (mg): 0
Diabetic exchange: 1 starch/bread; 1½ fruit

Tiramisu

This popular Italian dessert is both rich and beautiful. Try this easy yet impressive version.

1 C	skim milk	250 mL
1 T	butter or margarine	15 mL
1½ T	cornstarch	23 mL
1 T	sugar	15 mL
3 large	egg yolks, mixed lightly	3 large
2 t	vanilla extract	10 mL
1½ C	fat-free ricotta cheese or fat-free cottage cheese	375 mL
2 C	frozen low-fat non-dairy whipped topping, thawed	500 mL
¼ C	strong espresso, cooled	60 mL
¼ C	coffee liqueur	60 mL

| 1 | angel food cake | 1 |
| 2 C | fresh raspberries, or frozen, thawed | 500 mL |

Warm the milk and butter in a heavy-bottom medium saucepan or the top of a double boiler, stirring constantly. In a small bowl, mix together the cornstarch, sugar, and egg yolks. Blend well. Add the vanilla and blend. Transfer the egg mixture to the warm milk. Continue to heat and mix with a wire whisk until the mixture is thick. Look for whisk patterns, which indicate that it's done. Cool. Put the cheese into a mixing bowl. Beat at high speed with an electric mixer for 3–4 minutes. Add the cooled mixture and beat the two together at a low speed until well mixed. Fold in the whipped topping until thoroughly blended. In a small bowl, stir together the espresso and liqueur.

Using a sharp knife, cut the angel food cake crosswise into three layers. Put one layer into the bottom of a serving bowl. Brush with the espresso-liqueur mixture. Turn the layer over and brush the other side. Spoon one-third of the milk-cheese mixture over the cake. Arrange one-third of the raspberries around edges. Brush one side of another angel food cake layer and put it (brushed-side-down) in the bowl. Brush the top and spoon on one-third of the milk-cheese mixture and raspberries. Repeat the process for the last layer. Pour any remaining espresso liqueur on top of the third layer. Smooth the top and cover tightly. Refrigerate for at least 6 hours or up to 2 days before serving.

Yield: 12 servings
Each serving contains:
Calories (Kcal): 242   Total fat (g): 3
Carbohydrates (g): 43   Protein (g): 8
Sodium (mg): 295   Cholesterol (mg): 59
Diabetic exchange: 3 starch/bread

Strawberry Charlotte

This charlotte is layered angel food cake filled with pudding and strawberry preserves. If the preserves are too rigid to spread, add a little hot water and mix well. This should soften them up.

1	angel food cake	1
⅓ C	fruit-only strawberry preserves	80 mL
1 recipe	Vanilla Tart Filling (p. 45), or sugar-free low-fat strawberry pudding from a 4-serving package, made with skim milk according to package directions	1 recipe

Slice the angel food cake crosswise into three sections. Lay the bottom part, cut-side-up, on a serving plate. Spread with one-third of the jam. Prepare the tart filling and then spoon one-third of the vanilla filling or pudding evenly on top of the jam layer. Spread jam on top of the next layer of angel food cake and place it on top of the pudding layer. Repeat, ending with pudding on top. Refrigerate until serving.

Yield: 12 servings
Each serving contains:
Calories (Kcal): 196   Total fat (g): 3
Carbohydrates (g): 39   Protein (g): 5
Sodium (mg): 296   Cholesterol (mg): 23
Diabetic exchange: 1½ starch/bread; 1 fruit

Peach Charlotte

A taste of Georgia. Use fresh peaches instead of canned, if you have them, for the most authentic charlotte of all.

1	angel food cake	1
⅓ C	fruit-only peach preserves	80 mL
1 recipe	Vanilla Tart Filling (p. 45) or sugar-free low-fat vanilla pudding from a 4-serving package, made with skim milk according to package directions	1 recipe
15 oz	canned peaches, sliced, packed in juice without sugar, drained and chopped	425 g

Slice the angel food cake crosswise into three sections. Place the bottom part, cut-side-up, onto a serving plate. Prepare the tart filling. Spread the cut side of the cake on the plate with one-third of the jam. Mix the vanilla filling with the drained, chopped peaches. Spoon one-third of this mixture onto the first layer of the cake. Spread jam on top of the next layer of the cake and repeat, ending with pudding. Refrigerate until serving time.

Yield: 12 servings
Each serving contains:

Calories (Kcal): 211 — Total fat (g): 3
Carbohydrates (g): 43 — Protein (g): 5
Sodium (mg): 296 — Cholesterol (mg): 23
Diabetic exchange: 2 starch/bread; 1 fruit; ½ fat

Chocolate Charlotte

I've made this several different ways. In a pinch I use the pudding mix and whichever fruit preserves I have enough of. The raspberry-chocolate combination is the one you'd expect in an expensive restaurant.

1	angel food cake	1
⅓ C	fruit-only cherry preserves or seedless raspberry fruit-only preserves	80 mL
1 recipe	Chocolate Tart Filling (pp. 44–45), or sugar-free low-fat chocolate pudding from a package, made with skim milk according to package directions.	1 recipe

Follow the directions for Strawberry Charlotte, above.

Yield: 12 servings
Each serving contains:

Calories (Kcal): 190 — Total fat (g): 0.4
Carbohydrates (g): 43 — Protein (g): 5
Sodium (mg): 298 — Cholesterol (mg): 1
Diabetic exchange: ½ milk; 2 fruit

Jamaican Trifle

Taste this to see if the rum flavor is strong enough for you, and add more if you like. This is a buffet-table favorite.

15 oz	crushed pineapple, packed in juice, with no sugar added	420 g
1 T	rum extract	15 mL
1	angel food cake	1
2 C	frozen low-fat non-dairy whipped topping, thawed	500 mL

Drain the crushed pineapple, reserving the juice. Measure out ½ cup (125 mL) of the juice. Put it in a small bowl and mix in the rum extract. Slice the angel food cake into three layers. Brush the bottom of the bottom layer with the juice mixture and place it in a trifle bowl or other glass serving bowl. Brush the top of this layer with the juice. Spoon one-third of the pineapple on top of this layer. Brush the bottom of the next layer. Repeat, using all the juice and the rest of the crushed pineapple. Cover tightly and refrigerate for at least 6 hours. When serving, scoop a dollop of white topping onto each piece.

> Yield: 12 servings
> Each serving contains:
>
> | | |
> |---|---|
> | Calories (Kcal): 177 | Total fat (g): 1 |
> | Carbohydrates (g): 37 | Protein (g): 3.2 |
> | Sodium (mg): 253 | Cholesterol (mg): 0 |
>
> Diabetic exchange: 1 starch/bread; 1½ fruit

Individual Strawberry Trifles

These look especially elegant in tall, clear glasses.

2 C	fresh whole strawberries or frozen (no sugar), sliced (reserve ½ C whole for garnish)	500 mL
2 T	Grand Marnier liqueur	30 mL
1½ C	skim milk	375 mL
1 C	egg substitute or 4 eggs, slightly beaten	250 mL
1 t	vanilla extract	5 mL
4 pkgs.	saccharin or acesulfame-K sugar substitute	4 pkgs.
½	angel food cake, cut into 8 pieces	½
1¼ C	frozen low-fat non-dairy whipped topping, slightly softened	310 mL

In a small bowl, toss the sliced strawberries with the Grand Marnier. Cover and refrigerate. In the top of a double boiler over boiling water, scald the milk. Put the lightly beaten eggs in a small bowl. Pour about ½ C (125 mL) of the hot milk on top of the eggs, stirring constantly. Pour this mixture into the top of a double boiler. With only simmering water, and being sure the top pan does not come into contact with the water, cook, stirring constantly. When the custard is finished, it will easily coat a metal spoon. Remove the custard from over the water. Stir in the extract and sugar substitute.

When ready to assemble, put the custard into a medium mixing bowl and gently but thoroughly fold in the whipped topping. Tear off half of each of the eight pieces of angel food cake and push the half to the bottom of a tall parfait glass. Distribute half the strawberries over the pieces of angel food cake. Distribute half the custard in a similar fashion. Repeat with the other half pieces of angel food cake, strawberries, and custard. Cover tightly with plastic wrap and refrigerate until serving time, at least 2 hours. Garnish with the reserved strawberries.

Yield: 8 servings
Each serving contains:

Calories (Kcal): 202	Total fat (g): 4
Carbohydrates (g): 33	Protein (g): 7
Sodium (mg): 247	Cholesterol (mg): 107

Diabetic exchange: 2 starch/bread; 1 fat

Lemony Angel Food

The perfect solution for leftover angel food cake that is getting stale. The topping revives the cake.

½	angel food cake, cut into 6 pieces	½
1 pkg.	sugar-free lemon pudding mix	1 pkg.
(4 servings)	(prepared according to package directions)	(4 servings)
1¼ C	water or skim milk	310 mL
1 t	lemon juice	5 mL
1 recipe	Lemon Sauce (recipe follows)	1 recipe
½ C	frozen low-fat non-dairy whipped topping (optional)	125 mL

Cut each of the six pieces of cake into chunks and arrange them in six serving dishes. Mix the lemon pudding, made with water or skim milk, with the lemon juice and spoon over the angel food cake. Drizzle Lemon Sauce over the mixture. Top with a dollop of white topping, if desired.

> Yield: 6 servings
> Each serving contains:
>
> | | |
> |---|---|
> | Calories (Kcal): 149 | Total fat (g): 1 |
> | Carbohydrates (g): 35 | Protein (g): 4 |
> | Sodium (mg): 304 | Cholesterol (mg): 35 |
> | Diabetic exchange: 1 starch/bread; 1½ fruit | |

Lemon Sauce

This lemon sauce is best when used in a day or two. Keep it refrigerated.

⅓ C	fresh lemon juice	80 mL
6 pkgs.	saccharin or acesulfame-K sugar substitute	6 pkgs.
1 large	egg or equivalent egg substitute	1 large
1 T	cornstarch	15 mL
1 T	water	15 mL
1 t	vanilla extract	5 mL
1 t	aspartame sweetener	5 mL

Combine the lemon juice and saccharin or acesulfame-K in a saucepan over medium heat. Bring to a simmer. In a medium mixing bowl, beat the egg. Using a fork, blend together the cornstarch and water in a cup. Add this to the egg. Add a small amount of the lemon juice mixture to the egg mixture. Now put this into the saucepan with the remaining lemon mixture. Cook over medium heat, stirring constantly until thickened. Remove from heat. Cool. Stir in the vanilla and aspartame.

Yield: ⅔ C, or 6 servings
Each serving contains:
Calories (Kcal): 27   Total fat (g): 0.8
Carbohydrates (g): 4   Protein (g): 1
Sodium (mg): 15   Cholesterol (mg): 35
Diabetic exchange: free

Strawberries Chantilly

Don't forget to let the strawberries stand. That's the secret of getting them juicy.

2 C	fresh strawberries or frozen (no sugar), thawed	500 mL
1 T	sugar	15 mL
1 T	Kirsch or cherry liqueur (optional)	15 mL
1 C	frozen low-fat non-dairy whipped topping, thawed	250 mL
⅓	angel food cake	⅓

Cut the strawberries in half. In a mixing bowl, combine the strawberries, sugar, and liqueur, if you are using it. Let stand ½ hour to 1 hour. Just before serving fold together the strawberries and the whipped topping. Put one slice of angel food cake on each of four dessert plates. Spoon the strawberry mixture on top.

Yield: 4 servings
Each serving contains:
Calories (Kcal): 202   Total fat (g): 2
Carbohydrates (g): 41   Protein (g): 3
Sodium (mg): 254   Cholesterol (mg): 0
Diabetic exchange: 1 starch/bread; 2 fruit

Baked Goodies

Deep Dish Pie Shell

My husband, Chuck, experimented with the new fat-free butter and oil replacement product and got great results with this recipe.

2 C	flour	500 mL
11 T	fat-free butter and oil replacement product	165 mL
3–4 T	ice water	45–60 mL

Put the flour into a bowl. Using two knives or a pastry blender, cut in the butter and oil replacement until the mixture resembles coarse meal. Add about two tablespoons (30 mL) of water and work it in gently with a fork. Gradually add the ice water a little at a time, using fingers or a fork to work the dough into a ball. Don't let the ball become sticky, the result of too much water. Chill the dough for 30 minutes. On a lightly floured surface, flatten the dough into a circle with roundish edges or rectangular edges, depending on your deep dish pie pan.

With a rolling pin, roll the dough slightly larger than the pan, rolling from the center outward, the thinner the better. Fold the dough in half and gently lift it onto a pie pan coated with non-stick vegetable spray, being careful not to stretch it. Unfold the dough and pat it gently into the pan. Using a kitchen knife, cut away any dough that extends more than ¾ inch (3 cm) beyond the edge of the pan. Fold the outside dough over to make a double thickness around the rim of the pan. Press the edge down with a fork, or use your fingers to make a fluted edge. If the crust will be baked without any filling, prick the crust all over with a fork. Bake in 425°F (220°C) oven for approximately 12 to 15 minutes or until it looks as brown as you would like, or follow the directions of the recipe contained with the filling recipe.

Yield: 1 Deep Dish Pie Shell, or 8 servings
Each serving contains:
Calories (Kcal): 162   Total fat (g): 0.2
Carbohydrates (g): 36   Protein (g): 3
Sodium (mg): 8   Cholesterol (mg): 0
Diabetic exchange: 1 starch/bread; 1 fruit

Sweet Potato Pie

Rich and satisfying, a great dessert for a light meal.

1	frozen pie crust, unbaked, or Deep Dish Pie Shell, unbaked (p. 126)	1
3 large	sweet potatoes, peeled, cooked, well drained and mashed	3 large
¼ C	sugar	60 mL
6 pkgs.	saccharin	6 pkgs.
2 T	butter or margarine, melted	30 mL
1 t	cinnamon	5 mL
1 t	nutmeg	5 mL
1 t	allspice	5 mL
1 C	skim milk	250 mL
4 large	eggs or equivalent egg substitute, slightly beaten	4 large
1 t	vanilla	5 mL

Use a frozen pie crust or freeze a deep dish pie crust for 30 minutes. In a large bowl, combine the sweet potatoes, sugar, sugar substitute, butter, cinnamon, nutmeg, and allspice. Mix well. In another bowl, combine the remaining ingredients. Pour this wet mixture onto the sweet potato mixture. Mix well to combine. Pour this mixture into the pie crust. Put the pie in a 375°F (180°C) oven for 45–50 minutes. Test the pie for doneness by inserting a knife in the center. The pie is done when the knife comes out clean.

Yield: 8 servings

Each serving contains:

Calories (Kcal): 236   Total fat(g): 11

Carbohydrates(g): 29   Protein (g): 6

Sodium (mg): 188   Cholesterol (mg): 114

Diabetic exchange: 2 starch/bread; 2 fat

Squash Pie

This tastes like coconut custard. If the top is brown but the center isn't cooked, cover the pie with aluminum foil and bake for a few minutes more.

2 C	yellow squash, freshly grated, peeled	500 mL
¼ C	sugar	60 mL
6 pkgs.	saccharin or acesulfame-K sugar substitute	6 pkgs.
1 t	cornstarch	5 mL
1 t	vanilla	5 mL
2 t	coconut extract	10 mL
1 T	flour	15 mL
3 large	eggs or equivalent egg substitute, slightly beaten	3 large
¼ C	butter or margarine, melted	60 mL
1	Deep Dish Pie Shell, unbaked (p. 126)	1

In a large mixing bowl, combine all the ingredients except the pie shell, and mix well. Pour into the unbaked pie shell. Put the pie into a preheated 400°F (200°C) oven for 10–15 minutes. Reduce the temperature to 350°F (180°C) for 40–50 minutes until the top is golden brown.

> Yield: 8 slices
> Each slice contains:
> Calories (Kcal): 280   Total fat (g): 4
> Carbohydrates (g): 46   Protein (g): 6
> Sodium (mg): 93   Cholesterol (mg): 95
> Diabetic exchange: 2 starch/bread; 1 fruit; 1 fat

Blueberry Sour Cream Pie

I have used both fresh and frozen blueberries and they work equally well in this pie.

2 C	fresh or frozen blueberries	500 mL
1	frozen pie crust, unbaked, or Deep Dish Pie Shell, unbaked (p. 126)	1
1 C	fat-free sour cream	250 mL
2 T	sugar	30 mL
3 pkgs.	saccharin or acesulfame-K sugar substitute	3 pkgs.
1 large	egg yolk, lightly beaten	1 large
1 t	vanilla	1 t

Put the blueberries in the crust. Mix all the other ingredients in a mixing bowl. Pour this mixture over the blueberries. Bake in a preheated 375°F (190°C) oven for 45 minutes. The pie top will be lightly browned. Cool and chill before serving.

Yield: 8 servings
Each serving contains:

Calories (Kcal): 143	Total fat (g): 6
Carbohydrates (g): 19	Protein (g): 2
Sodium (mg): 132	Cholesterol (mg): 27

Diabetic exchange: 1 starch/bread; 1 fat

Quick Custard Pie

Cut down the fat by using egg substitute. I love this for winter nights.

4 large	eggs or equivalent egg substitute	4 large
3 T	sugar	45 mL
6 pkgs.	saccharin or acesulfame-K sugar substitute	6 pkgs.
¼ t	nutmeg	2 mL
1 t	vanilla extract	5 mL
½ t	butter extract	3 mL
1	unbaked pie crust, or Deep-Dish Pie Shell, unbaked (p. 126)	1

Put all the ingredients (except the pie shell!) into a blender or food processor. Process at a low speed until the sugar is dissolved and the mixture is well blended. Pour into the pie shell. Bake in a preheated 350°F (180°C) oven for 30 minutes or until a knife inserted into the center of the pie comes out clean.

Yield: 8 servings
Each serving contains:

Calories (Kcal): 160	Total fat (g): 9
Carbohydrates (g): 16	Protein (g): 4
Sodium (mg): 180	Cholesterol (mg): 106

Diabetic exchange: 1 starch/bread; 2 fat

Sour Cream Pie

Try serving this pie with raspberry or lemon sauce.

2 large	eggs or equivalent egg substitute	2 large
1 C	fat-free sour cream	250 mL
½ C	raisins	125 mL
2 T	sugar	30 mL
6 pkgs.	saccharin or acesulfame-K sugar substitute	6 pkgs.
1½ t	cinnamon	8 mL
¼ C	pecans, chopped fine optional)	60 mL
1	frozen pie crust, unbaked, or Deep Dish Pie Shell, unbaked (p. 126)	1

Put all the ingredients except the pecans and the pie crust in a blender or food processor. Process at medium speed until well mixed. Scrape the sides a few times, if necessary. Add the pecans if you're using them, and pulse a few times to blend. Pour into the pie shell. Bake in a preheated 450°F (230°C) oven for 15 minutes. Reduce heat to 350°F (180°C) and bake an additional 30 minutes.

Yield: 8 servings
Each serving contains:

Calories (Kcal): 163	Total fat (g): 6
Carbohydrates (g): 22	Protein (g): 4
Sodium (mg): 147	Cholesterol (mg): 53
Diabetic exchange: 1½ starch/bread; 1 fat	

Langues de Chat

My grandmother served these with coffee on her sunporch on summer afternoons. I've changed the recipe, but the wonderful rich character remains.

2 T	butter or margarine	30 mL
2 T	fat-free cream cheese	30 mL
3 pkgs.	acesulfame-K sugar substitute	3 pkgs.
3 T	sugar	45 mL
1 large	egg or equivalent egg substitute, lightly beaten	1 large
1 t	vanilla extract	5 mL
¼ t	butter extract	2 mL
½ C	flour, sifted	125 mL

In a medium bowl, beat the butter, cream cheese, acesulfame-K, and sugar until light and fluffy. Slowly beat in the egg and the two extracts. Fold in the flour to make a soft dough. Spoon the dough carefully into a pastry bag fitted with a 3/8" (1 cm) plain tip. Squeeze out 3" (7.5 cm) lengths onto greased baking sheets that have been lined with parchment or waxed paper. Cut off the dough with a sharp knife in between the cookies. Bake in a pre-heated 425°F (220°C) oven for 8–10 minutes, until the edges are lightly browned. Cool the sheets on a wire rack before removing the cookies.

Yield: 30 cookies
Each cookie contains:

Calories (Kcal): 23	Total fat (g): 1
Carbohydrates (g): 3	Protein (g): 1
Sodium (mg): 14	Cholesterol (mg): 9
Diabetic exchange: free	

Chocolate Mayonnaise Cake

This would have been loaded with fat before fat-free mayonnaise. It's a moist, rich chocolate cake.

2 C	sifted flour	500 mL
¼ C	sugar	60 mL
6 pkgs.	saccharin or acesulfame-K sugar substitute	6 pkgs.
1½ t	baking soda	8 mL
4 T	unsweetened cocoa powder	60 mL
1 C	cold water	250 mL
1 C	fat-free mayonnaise	250 mL

Mix together the dry ingredients in a large mixing bowl. In another bowl, beat together the cold water and mayonnaise. Add the water mixture to the dry ingredients. Mix well to combine. Prepare an 8 × 12" (20 × 30 cm) sheet cake pan, coating it with non-stick cooking spray. Pour the batter into the pan and bake it in a preheated 350°F (180°C) oven for 45 minutes or until a tester comes out clean. Cut into eight sections.

Yield: 8 pieces
Each piece contains:

Calories (Kcal): 147	Total fat (g): 0.7
Carbohydrates (g): 32	Protein (g): 4
Sodium (mg): 241	Cholesterol (mg): 0
Diabetic exchange: 1 starch/bread; 1 fruit	

Rich Lemon Shorties

For the calories, these are delicious. It's worth using potato flour for its smooth texture.

Base

½ C	fat-free cream cheese	125 mL
½ C	butter or margarine	125 mL
2 T	sugar	30 mL
3 pkgs.	acesulfame-K sugar substitute	3 pkgs.
2 C	flour	500 mL
½ C	potato flour	125 mL

Topping

2 T	lemon peel, freshly grated	30 mL
3 T	sugar	45 mL
3 pkgs.	acesulfame-K sugar substitute	3 pkgs.
3 large	eggs or equivalent egg substitute	3 large
½ C	sifted flour	125 mL
¾ t	baking powder	4 mL
3 T	lemon juice	45 mL
½ t	sugar (optional)	3 mL

Using an electric mixer, cream together the cream cheese, butter, sugar, and acesulfame-K. In another bowl, sift together the two flours. Add the flour mixture to the cream cheese mixture. Mix. With your hands, spread the mixture along the bottom of a 9×13" (23×33cm) lasagna pan. Refrigerate while you preheat a 350°F (180°C) oven. Bake 15–20 minutes. Base will be lightly browned. Cool on a wire rack.

Beat the lemon peel, sugar, acesulfame-K, and eggs until smooth and creamy. Sift the flour and baking powder together into a small bowl. Fold the sifted ingredients into the egg mixture. Stir in the lemon juice. Pour the mixture over a cooled base. Bake in a 350°F (180°C) oven for 25 minutes. Cool on a wire rack. Cut into squares. Sprinkle with the remaining sugar, if desired.

Yield: 30 squares
Each square contains:

Calories (Kcal): 95	Total fat (g): 4
Carbohydrates (g): 13	Protein (g): 2
Sodium (mg): 66	Cholesterol (mg): 30
Diabetic exchange: 1 starch/bread; ½ fat	

Cherry Cheese Suzette

Rich and sweet. A brunch favorite.

Batter

¼ C	fat-free butter and oil replacement product	60 mL
2 large	eggs or equivalent egg substitute	2 large
1¼ C	flour	310 mL
1 t	baking powder	5 mL
¾ C	skim milk	185 mL

Filling

2 C	fat-free cottage cheese	500 mL
1 t	butter extract	5 mL
1 pkg.	saccharin or acesulfame-K sugar substitute	1 pkg.
½ C	fruit-only cherry preserves	125 mL

Put the butter replacement in the mixing bowl of an electric mixer. Add the eggs and beat until smooth. In another bowl, combine the flour and baking powder. With mixer running at low speed, add the flour mixture to the egg mixture alternately with the milk. Blend for two minutes at low speed. Coat an 8" (20 cm) pan with non-stick cooking spray. Spoon half the batter into the pan. In a mixing bowl, combine the cottage cheese, butter extract, and sugar substitute. Pour the filling over the batter. Spread so the filling is evenly distributed. Dot with cherry filling. Carefully pour the remaining batter on top. Bake in a preheated 350°F (180°C) oven for 50–60 minutes. The top will be lightly browned.

Yield: 9 servings
Each serving contains:
Calories (Kcal): 164   Total fat (g): 1
Carbohydrates (g): 29   Protein (g): 10
Sodium (mg): 201   Cholesterol (mg): 52
Diabetic exchange: 2 starch/bread

Carrot Cake with Cream Cheese Icing

I made this carrot cake to taste as much as possible like those served at the old Commissary Restaurant in Philadelphia, my absolute favorite carrot cake.

2 C	flour	500 mL
2 t	cinnamon	10 mL
1 t	baking powder	5 mL
⅓ C	fat-free butter and oil replacement product	80 mL
4 T	sugar	60 mL
6 pkgs.	saccharin or acesulfame-K sugar substitute	6 pkgs.
3 large	eggs or egg substitute	3 large
3 medium	carrots, grated	3 medium
½ C	finely chopped walnuts (optional)	125 mL
1 recipe	Cream Cheese Icing (p. 135)	1 recipe

In a medium mixing bowl, blend together the flour, cinnamon, and baking powder. In another bowl, beat together the butter replacement, sugar, and sugar substitute. Beat in the eggs, one at a time, alternating with the flour mixture. Stir in the carrots and walnuts, if you are using them. Pour the batter into a 9" (14 cm) cake pan coated with non-stick vegetable spray. Bake in a 350°F (180°C) oven for 40 minutes. Cool the cake on a wire rack for 10 minutes before removing it from the pan. Ice with cream cheese frosting.

If cut into 8 servings, each serving contains:
Calories (Kcal): 250   Total fat (g): 2
Carbohydrates (g): 47   Protein (g): 8
Sodium (mg): 223   Cholesterol (mg): 85
Diabetic exchange: 2 starch/bread; 1 vegetable; 1 fruit

If cut into 10 servings, each serving contains:
Calories (Kcal): 200   Total fat (g): 2
Carbohydrates (g): 38   Protein (g): 6
Sodium (mg): 179   Cholesterol (mg): 68
Diabetic exchange: 2 starch/bread; ½ fruit

Cream Cheese Icing

Decadent!

¼ C	fat-free butter and oil replacement product	60 mL
8 oz	fat-free cream cheese	225 g
3 pkgs.	aspartame sweetener	3 pkgs.
2 t	vanilla extract	10 mL

Beat together all the ingredients until they are smoothly blended.

Yield: ¾ C (185 mL), or 8 or 10 servings

For 8 servings, each serving contains:

Calories (Kcal): 45	Total fat (g): 0
Carbohydrates (g): 7	Protein (g): 2
Sodium (mg): 138	Cholesterol (mg): 5
Diabetic exchange: ½ starch/bread	

For 10 servings, each serving contains:

Calories (Kcal): 0	Total fat(g): 0
Carbohydrates (g): 4	Protein (g): 1
Sodium (mg): 110	Cholesterol (mg): 4
Diabetic exchange: free	

Orange-Glazed Coffee Cake

Perfect for brunch.

1 pkg.	active dry yeast	1 pkg.
¼ C	warm water	60 mL
½ C	warm skim milk, 105–115°F (40–45°C)	125 mL
½ C	fresh orange juice, at room temperature	125 mL
3 T	sugar	45 mL
½ C	fat-free ricotta cheese	125 mL
1 T	orange peel, grated	15 mL
½ t	salt	3 mL
1 large	egg or equivalent egg substitute, lightly beaten	1 large
3½ C	flour (up to 4 cups)	875 mL
2–3 drops	oil	2–3 drops
1 recipe	Orange Icing (p. 137)	1 recipe

Put the yeast in a large mixing bowl. Add the warm water and stir. Set aside for 5–10 minutes. The mixture will become foamy. Add all the remaining ingredients except the flour, oil, and icing, and mix together to blend.

By hand or with a heavy duty electric mixer, beat in 2½ cups (625 mL) of the flour, a little at a time. The dough will become stiff. Use a handful of the remaining flour to coat a work board. Turn the batter onto the floured board. Adding more flour as the dough becomes sticky, knead the dough until it becomes smooth and elastic. This will take about 10 minutes.

Put a few drops of oil in the bottom of a large mixing bowl. Put the dough in the bowl and turn it over so it is coated with oil. Cover loosely with a damp dishcloth—damp, not wet. Let the dough rise in a warm place for 2 hours or until doubled. Punch down and knead again for a few minutes on the floured board.

Divide the dough into three equal parts. Use your hands to roll the pieces into three 20" (45 cm) strands. Braid. Arrange the braid in a 10" (25 cm) round cheesecake or springform pan. Cover with the damp cloth once again and let rise until doubled.

Bake in a preheated 425°F (220°C) oven for 25–30 minutes. Use a sharp knife to loosen the coffee cake from the pan. Remove the cake and cool on a wire rack. Spread Orange Icing on the cake while it is still somewhat warm. This is best served warm.

Yield: 12 servings

Each serving contains:

Calories (Kcal): 196   Total fat (g): 0.9

Carbohydrates (g): 39   Protein (g): 6

Sodium (mg): 108   Cholesterol (mg): 19

Diabetic exchange: 2 starch/bread; ½ fruit

Orange Icing

Especially for orange coffee cake or cupcakes.

¼ C	fruit-only marmalade preserves	60 mL
1 t	Triple Sec or orange extract	5 mL
½ C	orange juice	125 mL

Mix all the ingredients together in a small saucepan. Heat gently, stirring constantly until blended.

Yield: ¾ C (375 mL), or 12 servings

Each serving contains:

Calories (Kcal): 18   Total fat (g): 0

Carbohydrates (g): 4   Protein (g): 0.1

Sodium (mg): 0   Cholesterol (mg): 0

Diabetic exchange: free

Cupcakes with a Cherry on Top

Either orange or cream cheese icing can be used, depending on your preference.

1 C	flour	250 mL
1 pkg.	sugar-free vanilla pudding mix	1 pkg.
(4 servings)	(not instant)	(4 servings)
1¼ C	water or skim milk	310 mL
1½ t	baking powder	8 mL
3 T	fat-free butter and oil replacement product	45 mL
2 large	eggs or equivalent egg substitute	2 large
1 t	vanilla extract	5 mL
½ C	skim milk	125 mL
1 recipe	Orange Icing (p. 137)	1 recipe
	or Cream Cheese Frosting (p. 135)	
16	whole maraschino cherries	16

Combine flour, pudding mix, water or skim milk, and baking powder in a mixing bowl. Beat in the butter replacement, eggs, and vanilla extract. Beat for 1 minute. Beat in the milk. Fill muffin tins lined with paper baking cups two-thirds full. Bake in a preheated 350°F (180°C) oven for 15–17 minutes. Frost with Orange Icing or Cream Cheese Frosting and a maraschino cherry.

Yield: 16 cupcakes
Each cupcake contains:

Calories (Kcal): 72	Total fat (g): 0.8
Carbohydrates (g): 14	Protein (g): 2
Sodium (mg): 63	Cholesterol (mg): 27

Diabetic exchange: 1 starch/bread

Cream Cheese Pastries

Without the new fat-free dairy products, this recipe would have too much fat.

4 T	butter or margarine	60 mL
8 oz	fat-free cream cheese	225 g
2 T	sugar	30 mL
4 pkgs.	acesulfame-K sugar substitute	4 pkgs.
1 large	egg or equivalent egg substitute, lightly beaten	1 large
1½ C	flour	375 mL
1 t	baking powder	5 mL
½ t	butter extract	3 mL
½ C	fat-free sour cream	125 mL

In a large mixing bowl, cream the butter and cream cheese together until soft and creamy. Blend in the sugar and acesulfame-K. Blend in the egg. In another bowl, sift together the flour and baking powder. In a small bowl, mix together the butter extract and sour cream. In the large mixing bowl containing the butter and cream cheese, alternately add the flour mixture and the sour cream mixture. Blend thoroughly. Make a ball and wrap it in plastic wrap. Refrigerate until chilled. Roll dough on a lightly floured board until it is about ⅛" (3 mm) thick. Use cookie cutters to cut the dough into shapes. Place cookies on a baking sheet that has been coated with non-stick cooking spray. Bake in a preheated 400°F (200°C) oven for 8–10 minutes.

Yield: 90 (small) pastry cookies
Each cookie contains:
Calories (Kcal): 17   Total fat (g): 0.6
Carbohydrates (g): 2   Protein (g): 1
Sodium (mg): 23   Cholesterol (mg): 4
Diabetic exchange: free

Orange-Walnut Muffins

Be careful to handle the flour lightly as you measure, so you don't put in too much.

2 C	flour	500 mL
2 T	sugar	30 mL
1 T	baking powder	15 mL
1 C	water	250 mL
2 t	orange peel, grated	10 mL
1 t	orange extract	5 mL
½ t	butter extract	3 mL
2 large	egg whites	2 large
¼ C	finely chopped walnuts	60 mL
1 T	brown sugar	15 mL

In a large bowl, mix together the flour, sugar, and baking powder. Use a wire whisk to mix well. In another bowl, blend the water, orange peel, extracts, and egg whites. Pour on top of the dry ingredients. Stir lightly to moisten. Do not beat or over-stir. In a third bowl mix the walnuts and brown sugar. Spoon the batter into 12 muffin cups that have been coated with non-stick cooking spray. Top the muffins with the nut mixture. Bake in a preheated 400°F (200°C) oven for 14–16 minutes or until a tester inserted in the middle comes out clean. Cool the muffins on a wire rack before serving.

Yield: 12 Orange-Walnut Muffins
Each muffin contains:

Calories (Kcal): 107	Total fat (g): 2
Carbohydrates (g): 20	Protein (g): 3
Sodium (mg): 101	Cholesterol (mg): 0

Diabetic exchange: 1 starch/bread; ½ fat

Cherry Bread Pudding

A good way to use up slightly stale bread.

1 C	bread crumbs from 3 slices of Italian bread or 6 slices of French bread, toasted and then crumbled	250 mL
1 C	skim milk	250 mL
1 lb	ripe cherries, pitted	450 g
½ C	fruit-only cherry preserves (no added sugar)	125 mL
½ C	sliced almonds, toasted (optional)	125 mL
1 t	sugar	5 mL
1 C	fat-free sour cream	250 mL

Crumble the toast into a medium mixing bowl. Add the milk. Stir. Add the cherries and most of the almonds. Reserve a few tablespoons (about 30 mL) of almonds for topping. Coat a six-cup (1.5 L) baking dish with non-stick vegetable cooking spray. Pour the toast mixture into the prepared baking dish and top with the almonds, if you are using them. Sprinkle the teaspoon (5 mL) of sugar on top. Bake in a preheated 350°F (180°C) oven for 35–45 minutes. Serve each with a dollop of sour cream.

Yield: 6 servings
Each serving contains:

Calories (Kcal): 200	Total fat (g): 2
Carbohydrates (g): 40	Protein (g): 6
Sodium (mg): 181	Cholesterol (mg): 1

Diabetic exchange: 2 starch/bread; 1 fruit

Exchange Lists for Meal Planning

Y ou can make a difference in your blood glucose control through your food choices. You do not need special foods. In fact, the foods that are good for you are good for everyone.

If you have diabetes, it is important to eat about the same amount of food at the same time each day. Regardless of what your blood glucose level is, try not to skip meals or snacks. Skipping meals and snacks may lead to large swings in blood glucose levels.

To keep your blood glucose levels near normal, you need to balance the food you eat with the insulin your body makes or gets by injection and with your physical activities. Blood glucose monitoring gives you information to help you with this balancing act. Near-normal blood glucose levels help you feel better. And they may reduce or prevent the complications of diabetes.

The number of calories you need depends on your size, age, and activity level. If you are an adult, eating the right number of calories can help you reach and stay at a reasonable weight. Children and adolescents must eat enough calories so they grow and develop normally. Don't limit their calories to try to control blood glucose levels. Instead, adjust their insulin to cover the calories they need.

Of course, everyone needs to eat nutritious foods. Our good health depends on eating a variety of foods that contain the right amounts of carbohydrate, protein, fat, vitamins, minerals, fiber, and water.

What Are Carbohydrate, Protein, and Fat?

Carbohydrate, protein, and fat are found in the food you eat. They supply your body with energy, or calories. Your body needs insulin to use this energy. Insulin is made in the pancreas. If you have diabetes, either your pancreas is no longer making insulin or your body can't use the insulin it is making. In either case, your blood glucose levels are not normal.

Carbohydrate. Starch and sugar in foods are carbohydrates. Starch is in breads, pasta, cereals, potatoes, peas, beans, and lentils. Naturally present sugars are in fruits, milk, and vegetables. Added sugars are in desserts, candy, jams, and syrups. All of these carbohydrates provide 4 calories per gram and can affect your blood glucose levels.

When you eat carbohydrates, they turn into glucose and travel in your bloodstream. Insulin helps the glucose enter the cells, where it can be used for energy or stored. Eating the same amount of carbohydrate daily at meals and snacks helps you control your blood glucose levels.

Protein. Protein is in meats, poultry, fish, milk and other dairy products, eggs, and beans, peas, and lentils. Starches and vegetables also have small amounts of protein.

The body uses protein for growth, maintenance, and energy. Protein has 4 calories of energy per gram. Again, your body needs insulin to use the protein you eat.

Fat. Fat is in margarine, butter, oils, salad dressings, nuts, seeds, milk, cheese, meat, fish, poultry, snack foods, ice cream, and desserts.

There are different types of fat: monounsaturated, polyunsaturated, and saturated. Everyone should eat less of the saturated fats found in meats, dairy products, coconut, palm or palm kernel oil, and hardened shortenings. Saturated fats can raise your blood levels of cholesterol. The fats that are best are the monounsaturated fats found in canola oil, olive oil, nuts, and avocado. The polyunsaturated fats found in corn oil, soybean oil, or sunflower oil are also good choices.

After you eat fat, it travels in your bloodstream. You need insulin to store fat in the cells of your body. Fats are used for energy. In fact, fats have 9 calories per gram, more than two times the calories you get from carbohydrate and protein.

What Else Do I Need to Know?

Vitamins and Minerals. Most foods in the exchange lists are good sources of vitamins and minerals. If you eat a variety of these foods you probably do not need a vitamin or mineral supplement.

Salt or Sodium. High blood pressure may be made worse by eating too much sodium (salt and salty foods). Try to use less salt in cooking and at the table.

In the lists, foods that are high in sodium (400 milligrams or more of sodium per exchange) have a salt shaker symbol (▲).

Alcohol. You may have an alcoholic drink occasionally. If you take insulin or a diabetes pill, be sure to eat food with your drink. Ask your dietitian about a safe amount of alcohol for you and how to work it into your meal plan.

How Do I Know What to Eat and When?

You and your dietitian will work out a meal plan to get the right balance between your food, medication, and exercise.

The lists of food choices (exchange lists) can help you make interesting and healthy food choices. Exchange lists and a meal plan help you know what to eat, how much to eat, and when to eat.

There are three main groups—the Carbohydrate group, the Meat and Meat Substitute group (protein), and the Fat group. Starch, fruit, milk, other carbohydrates, and vegetables are in the Carbohydrate group. The Meat and Meat Substitute group is divided into very lean, lean, medium-fat, and high-fat foods. You can see at a glance which are the lower-fat choices. Foods in the Fat group—monounsaturated, polyunsaturated, and saturated—have very small serving sizes.

What Are Exchange Lists?

Exchange lists are foods listed together because they are alike. Each serving of a food has about the same amount of carbohydrate, protein, fat, and calories as the other foods on that list. That is why any food on a list can be "exchanged," or traded, for any other food on the same list. For example, you can trade the slice of bread you might eat for breakfast for one-half cup of cooked cereal. Each of these foods equals one starch choice.

Exchange Lists

Foods are listed with their serving sizes, which are usually measured after cooking. When you begin, you should measure the size of each serving. This may help you learn to "eyeball" correct serving sizes.

The following chart shows the amount of nutrients in one serving from each list.

Groups/Lists	Carbohydrate (grams)	Protein (grams)	Fat (grams)	Calories
Carbohydrate Group				
Starch	15	3	1 or less	80
Fruit	15	—	—	60
Milk				
Skim	12	8	0–3	90
Low-fat	12	8	5	120
Whole	12	8	8	150
Other carbohydrates	15	varies	varies	varies
Vegetables	5	2	—	25
Meat and Meat Substitute Group				
Very lean	—	7	0–1	35
Lean	—	7	3	55
Medium-fat	—	7	5	75
High-fat	—	7	8	100
Fat Group	—	—	5	45

The exchange lists provide you with a lot of food choices (foods from the basic food groups, foods with added sugars, free foods, combination foods, and fast foods). This gives you variety in your meals. Several foods, such as beans, peas, and lentils, bacon, and peanut butter, are on two lists. This gives you flexibility in putting your meals together. Whenever you choose new foods or vary your meal plan, monitor your blood glucose to see how these different foods affect your blood glucose level.

Most foods in the Carbohydrate group have about the same amount of carbohydrate per serving. You can exchange starch, fruit, or milk choices in your meal plan. Vegetables are in this group but contain only about 5 grams of carbohydrate.

A Word about Food Labels

Exchange information is based on foods found in grocery stores. However, food companies often change the ingredients in their products. That is why you need to check the Nutrition Facts panel of the food label.

The Nutrition Facts tell you the number of calories and grams of carbohydrate, protein, and fat in one serving. Compare these numbers with the exchange information to see how many exchanges you will be eating. In this way, food labels can help you add foods to your meal plans.

Ask your dietitian to help you use food label information to plan your meals.

Getting Started!

See your dietitian regularly when you are first learning how to use your meal plan and the exchange lists. Your meal plan can be adjusted to fit changes in your lifestyle, such as work, school, vacation, or travel. Regular nutrition counseling can help you make positive changes in your eating habits.

Careful eating habits will help you feel better and be healthier, too. Best wishes and good eating with *Exchange Lists for Meal Planning.*

Starch List

Cereals, grains, pasta, breads, crackers, snacks, starchy vegetables, and cooked beans, peas, and lentils are starches. In general, one starch is:

- 1/2 cup of cereal, grain, pasta, or starchy vegetable,
- 1 ounce of a bread product, such as 1 slice of bread,
- 3/4 to 1 ounce of most snack foods. (Some snack foods may also have added fat.)

Nutrition Tips

1. Most starch choices are good sources of B vitamins.
2. Foods made from whole grains are good sources of fiber.
3. Beans, peas, and lentils are a good source of protein and fiber.

Selection Tips

1. Choose starches made with little fat as often as you can.
2. Starchy vegetables prepared with fat count as one starch and one fat.
3. Bagels or muffins can be 2, 3, or 4 ounces in size, and can, therefore, count as 2, 3, or 4 starch choices. Check the size you eat.
4. Most of the serving sizes are measured after cooking.
5. Always check Nutrition Facts on the food label.

One starch exchange equals 15 grams carbohydrate, 3 grams protein, 0–1 grams fat, and 80 calories.

Bread		Cereals and Grains	
Bagel	1/2 (1 oz)	Bran cereals	1/2 cup
Bread, reduced-calorie	2 slices (1 1/2 oz)	Bulgur	1/2 cup
		Cereals	1/2 cup
Bread, white, whole-wheat, pumpernickel, rye	1 slice (1 oz)	Cereals, unsweetened, ready-to-eat	3/4 cup
Bread sticks, crisp, 4 in. long x 1/2 in.	2 (2/3 oz)	Cornmeal (dry)	3 Tbsp
		Couscous	1/3 cup
English muffin	1/2	Flour (dry)	3 Tbsp
Hot dog or hamburger bun	1/2 (1 oz)	Granola, low-fat	1/4 cup
Pita, 6 in. across	1/2	Grape-Nuts®	1/4 cup
Raisin bread, unfrosted	1 slice (1 oz)	Grits	1/2 cup
Roll, plain, small	1 (1 oz)	Kasha	1/2 cup
Tortilla, corn, 6 in. across	1	Millet	1/4 cup
Tortilla, flour, 7–8 in. across	1	Muesli	1/4 cup
Waffle, 4 1/2 in. square, reduced-fat	1	Oats	1/2 cup
		Pasta	1/2 cup

Puffed cereal	1 1/2 cups
Rice milk	1/2 cup
Rice, white or brown	1/3 cup
Shredded Wheat®	1/2 cup
Sugar-frosted cereal	1/2 cup
Wheat germ	3 Tbsp

Starchy Vegetables

Baked beans	1/3 cup
Corn	1/2 cup
Corn on cob, medium	1 (5 oz)
Mixed vegetables with corn, peas, or pasta	1 cup
Peas, green	1/2 cup
Plantain	1/2 cup
Potato, baked or boiled	1 small (3 oz)
Potato, mashed	1/2 cup
Squash, winter (acorn, butternut)	1 cup
Yam, sweet potato, plain	1/2 cup

Crackers and Snacks

Animal crackers	8
Graham crackers, 2 1/2 in. square	3
Matzoh	3/4 oz
Melba toast	4 slices
Oyster crackers	24
Popcorn (popped, no fat added or low-fat microwave)	3 cups
Pretzels	3/4 oz
Rice cakes, 4 in. across	2
Saltine-type crackers	6
Snack chips, fat-free (tortilla, potato)	15–20 (3/4 oz)
Whole-wheat crackers, no fat added	2–5 (3/4 oz)

Beans, Peas, and Lentils

(*Count as 1 starch exchange, plus 1 very lean meat exchange.*)

Beans and peas (garbanzo, pinto, kidney, white, split, black-eyed)	1/2 cup
Lima beans	2/3 cup
Lentils	1/2 cup
Miso ☙	3 Tbsp

Starchy Foods Prepared with Fat

(*Count as 1 starch exchange, plus 1 fat exchange.*)

Biscuit, 2 1/2 in. across	1
Chow mein noodles	1/2 cup
Corn bread, 2 in. cube	1 (2 oz)
Crackers, round butter type	6
Croutons	1 cup
French-fried potatoes	16–25 (3 oz)
Granola	1/4 cup
Muffin, small	1 (1 1/2 oz)
Pancake, 4 in. across	2
Popcorn, microwave	3 cups
Sandwich crackers, cheese or peanut butter filling	3
Stuffing, bread (prepared)	1/3 cup
Taco shell, 6 in. across	2
Waffle, 4 1/2 in. square	1
Whole-wheat crackers, fat added	4–6 (1 oz)

☙ = 400 mg or more of sodium per exchange.

Starches often swell in cooking, so a small amount of uncooked starch will become a much larger amount of cooked food. The following table shows some of the changes.

Food (Starch Group)	Uncooked	Cooked
Oatmeal	3 Tbsp	1/2 cup
Cream of wheat	2 Tbsp	1/2 cup
Grits	3 Tbsp	1/2 cup
Rice	2 Tbsp	1/3 cup
Spaghetti	1/4 cup	1/2 cup
Noodles	1/3 cup	1/2 cup
Macaroni	1/4 cup	1/2 cup
Dried beans	1/4 cup	1/2 cup
Dried peas	1/4 cup	1/2 cup
Lentils	3 Tbsp	1/2 cup

Fruit List

Fresh, frozen, canned, and dried fruits and fruit juices are on this list. In general, one fruit exchange is:

- 1 small to medium fresh fruit,
- 1/2 cup of canned or fresh fruit or fruit juice,
- 1/4 cup of dried fruit.

Nutrition Tips

1. Fresh, frozen, and dried fruits have about 2 grams of fiber per choice. Fruit juices contain very little fiber.
2. Citrus fruits, berries, and melons are good sources of vitamin C.

Selection Tips

1. Count 1/2 cup cranberries or rhubarb sweetened with sugar substitutes as free foods.
2. Read the Nutrition Facts on the food label. If one serving has more than 15 grams of carbohydrate, you will need to adjust the size of the serving you eat or drink.
3. Portion sizes for canned fruits are for the fruit and a small amount of juice.
4. Whole fruit is more filling than fruit juice and may be a better choice.
5. Food labels for fruits may contain the words "no sugar added" or "unsweetened." This means that no sucrose (table sugar) has been added.
6. Generally, fruit canned in extra light syrup has the same amount of carbohydrate per serving as the "no sugar added" or the juice pack. All canned fruits on the fruit list are based on one of these three types of pack.

One fruit exchange equals 15 grams carbohydrate and 60 calories. The weight includes skin, core, seeds, and rind.

Fruit	
Apple, unpeeled, small	1 (4 oz)
Applesauce, unsweetened	1/2 cup
Apples, dried	4 rings
Apricots, fresh	4 whole (5 1/2 oz)
Apricots, dried	8 halves
Apricots, canned	1/2 cup
Banana, small	1 (4 oz)
Blackberries	3/4 cup
Blueberries	3/4 cup
Cantaloupe, small	1/3 melon (11 oz)
	or 1 cup cubes
Cherries, sweet, fresh	12 (3 oz)
Cherries, sweet, canned	I/2 cup
Dates	3
Figs, fresh	1 1/2 large
	or 2 medium (3 1/2 oz)
Figs, dried	1 1/2
Fruit cocktail	1/2 cup
Grapefruit, large	1/2 (11 oz)
Grapefruit sections, canned	3/4 cup
Grapes, small	17 (3 oz)
Honeydew melon	1 slice (10 oz)
	or 1 cup cubes
Kiwi	1 (3 1/2 oz)
Mandarin oranges, canned	3/4 cup
Mango, small	1/2 fruit (5 1/2 oz)
	or 1/2 cup
Nectarine, small	1 (5 oz)

Orange, small	1 (6 1/2 oz)
Papaya	1/2 fruit (8 oz)
	or 1 cup cubes
Peach, medium, fresh	1 (6 oz)
Peaches, canned	1/2 cup
Pear, large, fresh	1/2 (4 oz)
Pears, canned	1/2 cup
Pineapple, fresh	3/4 cup
Pineapple, canned	1/2 cup
Plums, small	2 (5 oz)
Plums, canned	1/2 cup
Prunes, dried	3
Raisins	2 Tbsp
Raspberries	1 cup
Strawberries	1 1/4 cup whole berries
Tangerines, small	2 (8 oz)
Watermelon	1 slice (13 1/2 oz)
	or 1 1/4 cup cubes

Fruit Juice

Apple juice/cider	1/2 cup
Cranberry juice cocktail	1/3 cup
Cranberry juice cocktail, reduced-calorie	1 cup
Fruit juice blends, 100% juice	1/3 cup
Grape juice	1/3 cup
Grapefruit juice	1/2 cup
Orange juice	1/2 cup
Pineapple juice	1/2 cup
Prune juice	1/3 cup

Milk List

Different types of milk and milk products are on this list. Cheeses are on the Meat list and cream and other dairy fats are on the Fat list. Based on the amount of fat they contain, milks are divided into skim/very low-fat milk, low-fat milk, and whole milk. One choice of these includes:

	Carbohydrate (grams)	Protein (grams)	Fat (grams)	Calories
Skim/very low-fat	12	8	0–3	90
Low-fat	12	8	5	120
Whole	12	8	8	150

Nutrition Tips

1. Milk and yogurt are good sources of calcium and protein. Check the food label.
2. The higher the fat content of milk and yogurt, the greater the amount of saturated fat and cholesterol. Choose lower-fat varieties.
3. For those who are lactose intolerant, look for lactose-reduced or lactose-free varieties of milk.

Selection Tips

1. One cup equals 8 fluid ounces or 1/2 pint.
2. Look for chocolate milk, frozen yogurt, and ice cream on the Other Carbohydrates list.
3. Nondairy creamers are on the Free Foods list.
4. Look for rice milk on the Starch list.

One milk exchange equals 12 grams carbohydrate and 8 grams protein.

Skim and Very Low-fat Milk
(0–3 grams fat per serving)

Skim milk	1 cup
1/2% milk	1 cup
1% milk	1 cup
Nonfat or low-fat buttermilk	1 cup
Evaporated skim milk	1/2 cup
Nonfat dry milk	1/3 cup dry
Plain nonfat yogurt	3/4 cup
Nonfat or low-fat fruit-flavored yogurt sweetened with aspartame or with a nonnutritive sweetener	1 cup

Low-fat
(5 grams fat per serving)

2% milk	1 cup
Plain low-fat yogurt	3/4 cup
Sweet acidophilus milk	1 cup

Whole Milk
(8 grams fat per serving)

Whole milk	1 cup
Evaporated whole milk	1/2 cup
Goat's milk	1 cup
Kefir	1 cup

Vegetable List

Vegetables that contain small amounts of carbohydrates and calories are on this list. Vegetables contain important nutrients. Try to eat at least 2 or 3 vegetable choices each day. In general, one vegetable exchange is:

- 1/2 cup of cooked vegetables or vegetable juice,
- 1 cup of raw vegetables.

If you eat 1 to 2 vegetable choices at a meal or snack, you do not have to count the calories or carbohydrates because they contain small amounts of these nutrients.

Nutrition Tips

1. Fresh and frozen vegetables have less added salt than canned vegetables. Drain and rinse canned vegetables if you want to remove some salt.
2. Choose more dark green and dark yellow vegetables, such as spinach, broccoli, romaine, carrots, chilies, and peppers.
3. Broccoli, brussels sprouts, cauliflower, greens, peppers, spinach, and tomatoes are good sources of vitamin C.
4. Vegetables contain 1 to 4 grams of fiber per serving.

Selection Tips

1. A one-cup portion of broccoli is a portion about the size of a lightbulb.
2. Canned vegetables and juices are available without added salt.
3. If you eat more than 3 cups of raw vegetables or 1 1/2 cups of cooked vegetables at one meal, count them as 1 carbohydrate choice.
4. Starchy vegetables such as corn, peas, winter squash, and potatoes that contain larger amounts of calories and carbohydrates are on the Starch list.

**One vegetable exchange equals 5 grams carbohydrate,
2 grams protein, 0 grams fat, and 25 calories.**

Artichoke
Artichoke hearts
Asparagus
Beans (green, wax, Italian)
Bean sprouts
Beets
Broccoli
Brussels sprouts
Cabbage
Carrots
Cauliflower
Celery
Cucumber
Eggplant
Green onions or scallions
Greens (collard, kale, mustard, turnip)

Kohlrabi
Leeks
Mixed vegetables (without corn, peas, or pasta)
Mushrooms
Okra
Onions
Pea pods
Peppers (all varieties)
Radishes
Salad greens (endive, escarole, lettuce, romaine, spinach)
Sauerkraut ◣
Spinach

◣ = 400 mg or more sodium per exchange.

Summer squash
Tomato
Tomatoes, canned
Tomato sauce ✂.
Tomato/vegetable juice ✂.
Turnips

Water chestnuts
Watercress
Zucchini
✂. = 400 mg or more sodium per exchange.

Meat and Meat Substitutes List

Meat and meat substitutes that contain both protein and fat are on this list. In general, one meat exchange is:
- 1 ounce meat, fish, poultry, or cheese,
- 1/2 cup beans, peas, and lentils. Based on the amount of fat they contain, meats are divided into very lean, lean, medium-fat, and high-fat lists. This is done so you can see which ones contain the least amount of fat. One ounce (one exchange) of each of these includes:

	Carbohydrate (grams)	Protein (grams)	Fat (grams)	Calories
Very lean	0	7	0–1	35
Lean	0	7	3	55
Medium-fat	0	7	5	75
High-fat	0	7	8	100

Nutrition Tips
1. Choose very lean and lean meat choices whenever possible. Items from the high-fat group are high in saturated fat, cholesterol, and calories and can raise blood cholesterol levels.
2. Meats do not have any fiber.
3. Some processed meats, seafood, and soy products may contain carbohydrate when consumed in large amounts. Check the Nutrition Facts on the label to see if the amount is close to 15 grams. If so, count it as a carbohydrate choice as well as a meat choice.

Selection Tips
1. Weigh meat after cooking and removing bones and fat. Four ounces of raw meat is equal to 3 ounces of cooked meat. Some examples of meat portions are:
- 1 ounce cheese = 1 meat choice and is about the size of a one-inch cube
- 2 ounces meat = 2 meat choices, such as 1 small chicken leg or thigh or 1/2 cup cottage cheese or tuna
- 3 ounces meat = 3 meat choices and is about the size of a deck of cards, such as 1 medium pork chop, 1 small hamburger, 1/2 of a whole chicken breast, or 1 unbreaded fish fillet
2. Limit your choices from the high-fat group to three times per week or less.
3. Most grocery stores stock Select and Choice grades of meat. Select grades of meat are the leanest meats. Choice grades contain a moderate amount of fat, and Prime cuts of meat have the highest amount of fat. Restaurants usually

serve Prime cuts of meat.
4. "Hamburger" may contain added seasoning and fat, but ground beef does not.
5. Read labels to find products that are low in fat and cholesterol (5 grams or less of fat per serving).
6. Peanut butter, in smaller amounts, is also found on the Fats list.
7. Bacon, in smaller amounts, is also found on the Fats list.

Meal Planning Tips
1. Bake, roast, broil, grill, poach, steam, or boil these foods rather than frying.
2. Place meat on a rack so the fat will drain off during cooking.
3. Use a nonstick spray and a nonstick pan to brown or fry foods.
4. Trim off visible fat before or after cooking.
5. If you add flour, bread crumbs, coating mixes, fat, or marinades when cooking, ask your dietitian how to count it in your meal plan.

Lean Meat and Substitutes List

One exchange equals 0 grams carbohydrate, 7 grams protein, 3 grams fat, and 55 calories.

One lean meat exchange is equal to any one of the following items.

Beef: USDA Select or Choice grades of lean beef trimmed of fat, such as round, sirloin, and flank steak; tenderloin; roast (rib, chuck, rump); steak (T-bone, porterhouse, cubed); ground round   1 oz

Pork: Lean pork, such as fresh ham; canned, cured, or boiled ham; Canadian bacon ↖ ; tenderloin, center loin chop   1 oz

Lamb: Roast, chop, leg   1 oz

Veal: Lean chop, roast   1 oz

Poultry: Chicken, turkey (dark meat, no skin), chicken (white meat, with skin), domestic duck or goose (well-drained of fat, no skin)   1 oz

Fish:
Herring
(uncreamed or smoked)   1 oz
Oysters   6 medium

Salmon (fresh or canned), catfish   1 oz
Sardines (canned)   2 medium
Tuna (canned in oil, drained)   1 oz
Game: Goose (no skin), rabbit   1 oz
Cheese:
4.5%-fat cottage cheese   1/4 cup
Grated Parmesan   2 Tbsp
Cheeses with 3 grams or less fat per ounce   1 oz
Other:
Hot dogs with 3 grams or less fat per ounce ↖   1 1/2 oz
Processed sandwich meat with 3 grams or less fat per ounce, such as turkey pastrami or kielbasa   1 oz
Liver, heart (high in cholesterol)   1 oz

High-Fat Meat and Substitutes List

**One exchange equals 0 grams carbohydrate,
7 grams protein, 8 grams fat, and 100 calories.**

Remember that these items are high in saturated fat, cholesterol, and calories and may raise blood cholesterol levels if eaten on a regular basis.

One high-fat meat exchange is equal to any one of the following items.

Pork: Spareribs, ground pork,		chicken) ➤	1 (10/lb)
pork sausage	1 oz	Bacon	3 slices (20 slices/lb)
Cheese: All regular cheeses, such as		Count as one high-fat meat	
American ➤, Cheddar,		plus one fat exchange.	
Monterey Jack, Swiss	1 oz	Hot dog (beef, pork,	
Other: Processed sandwich meats with		or combination) ➤	1 (10/lb)
8 grams or less fat per ounce, such as		Peanut butter (contains	
bologna, pimento loaf, salami	1 oz	unsaturated fat)	2 Tbsp
Sausage, such as bratwurst, Italian,		➤ = 400 mg or more sodium per	
knockwurst, Polish, smoked	1 oz	exchange.	
Hot dog (turkey or			

Fat List

Fats are divided into three groups, based on the main type of fat they contain: monounsaturated, polyunsaturated, and saturated. Small amounts of monounsaturated and polyunsaturated fats in the foods we eat are linked with good health benefits. Saturated fats are linked with heart disease and cancer. In general, one fat exchange is:

- 1 teaspoon of regular margarine or vegetable oil,
- 1 tablespoon of regular salad dressings.

Nutrition Tips

1. All fats are high in calories. Limit serving sizes for good nutrition and health.
2. Nuts and seeds contain small amounts of fiber, protein, and magnesium.
3. If blood pressure is a concern, choose fats in the unsalted form to help lower sodium intake, such as unsalted peanuts.

Selection Tips

1. Check the Nutrition Facts on food labels for serving sizes. One fat exchange is based on a serving size containing 5 grams of fat.
2. When selecting regular margarines, choose those with liquid vegetable oil as the first ingredient. Soft margarines are not as saturated as stick margarines. Soft margarines are healthier choices. Avoid those listing hydrogenated or partially hydrogenated fat as the first ingredient.
3. When selecting low-fat margarines, look for liquid vegetable oil as the second ingredient. Water is usually the first ingredient.
4. When used in smaller amounts, bacon and peanut butter are counted as fat choices. When used in larger amounts, they are counted as high-fat meat choices.
5. Fat-free salad dressings are on the Free Foods list.

6. See the Free Foods list for nondairy coffee creamers, whipped topping, and fat-free products, such as margarines, salad dressings, mayonnaise, sour cream, cream cheese, and nonstick cooking spray.

Monounsaturated Fats List

(One fat exchange equals 5 grams fat and 45 calories.)

Avocado, medium	1/8 (1 oz)
Oil (canola, olive, peanut)	1 tsp
Olives: ripe (black)	8 large
green, stuffed ↖	10 large

Nuts

almonds, cashews	6 nuts
mixed (50% peanuts)	6 nuts
peanuts	10 nuts
pecans	4 halves
Peanut butter, smooth or crunchy	2 tsp
Sesame seeds	1 Tbsp
Tahini paste	2 tsp

Polyunsaturated Fats List

(One fat exchange equals 5 grams fat and 45 calories.)

Margarine: stick, tub, or squeeze	1 tsp
lower-fat	
(30% to 50% vegetable oil)	1 Tbsp
Mayonnaise: regular	1 tsp
reduced-fat	1 Tbsp
Nuts, walnuts, English	4 halves
Oil (corn, safflower, soybean)	1 tsp
Salad dressing: regular ↖	1 Tbsp
reduced-fat	2 Tbsp
Miracle Whip Salad Dressing®:	
regular	2 tsp
reduced-fat	1 Tbsp
Seeds: pumpkin, sunflower	1 Tbsp

Saturated Fats List*

(One fat exchange equals 5 grams fat and 45 calories.)

Bacon, cooked	1 slice (20 slices/lb)
Bacon, grease	1 tsp
Butter: stick	1 tsp
whipped	2 tsp
reduced-fat	1 Tbsp
Chitterlings, boiled	2 Tbsp (1/2 oz)
Coconut, sweetened, shredded	2 Tbsp
Cream, half and half	2 Tbsp
Cream cheese: regular	1 Tbsp (1/2 oz)
reduced-fat	2 Tbsp (1 oz)
Fatback or salt pork, see below	
Shortening or lard	1 tsp
Sour cream: regular	2 Tbsp
reduced-fat	3 Tbsp

Use a piece 1 in.×1 in.×1/4 in. if you plan to eat the fatback cooked with vegetables. Use a piece 2 in. x 1 in. x 1/2 in. when eating only the vegetables with the fatback removed.

*Saturated fats can raise blood cholesterol levels.

Free Foods List

A *free food* is any food or drink that contains less than 20 calories or less than 5 grams of carbohydrate per serving. Foods with a serving size listed should be limited to three servings per day. Be sure to spread them out throughout the day. If you eat all three servings at one time, it could affect your blood glucose level. Foods listed without a serving size may be eaten as often as you like.

Fat-free or Reduced-fat Foods

Cream cheese, fat-free	1 Tbsp
Creamers, nondairy, liquid	1 Tbsp
Creamers, nondairy, powdered	2 tsp
Mayonnaise, fat-free	1 Tbsp
Mayonnaise, reduced-fat	1 tsp
Margarine, fat-free	4 Tbsp
Margarine, reduced-fat	1 tsp
Miracle Whip®, nonfat	1 Tbsp
Miracle Whip®, reduced-fat	1 tsp
Nonstick cooking spray	
Salad dressing, fat-free	1 Tbsp
Salad dressing, fat-free, Italian	2 Tbsp
Salsa	1/4 cup
Sour cream, fat-free, reduced-fat	1 Tbsp
Whipped topping, regular or light	2 Tbsp

Sugar-free or Low-sugar Foods

Candy, hard, sugar-free	1 candy
Gelatin dessert, sugar-free	
Gelatin, unflavored	
Gum, sugar-free	
Jam or jelly, low-sugar or light	2 tsp
Sugar substitutes	
Syrup, sugar-free	2 Tbsp

Sugar substitutes, alternatives, or replacements that are approved by the Food and Drug Administration (FDA) are safe to use. Common brand names include: Equal® (aspartame), Sprinkle Sweet® (saccharin), Sweet One® (acesulfame K), Sweet-10® (saccharin), Sugar Twin®, (saccharin), Sweet 'n Low® (saccharin)

Drinks

Bouillon, broth, consommé ➤	
Bouillon or broth, low-sodium	
Carbonated or mineral water	
Club soda	
Cocoa powder, unsweetened	1 Tbsp
Coffee	
Diet soft drinks, sugar-free	
Drink mixes, sugar-free	
Tea	
Tonic water, sugar-free	

Condiments

Catsup	1 Tbsp
Horseradish	
Lemon juice	
Lime juice	
Mustard	
Pickles, dill ➤	1 1/2 large
Soy sauce, regular or light ➤	
Taco sauce	1 Tbsp
Vinegar	

Seasonings

Be careful with seasonings that contain sodium or are salts, such as garlic or celery salt, and lemon pepper.

Flavoring extracts
Garlic
Herbs, fresh or dried
Pimento
Spices
Tabasco® or hot pepper sauce
Wine, used in cooking
Worcestershire sauce

➤ = 400 mg or more of sodium per choice.

Index

A
angel food cake, 117-122
apple juice, 41
apples
  Apple Strudel Filling, 41
  Fried Spiced Apples, 20
apricot nectar
  Apricot Cream Pie, 86
apricot preserves
  Apricot Roll-Up, 68
apricots
  Apricot Cream Pie, 86
  Apricot Filling for Strudel, 42
Austrian Raspberry Cream Crêpes, 61
B
Baked Alaska-type dessert, 82, 83, 94
bananas
  Banana Cream and Strawberry Pie, 92-93
  Banana Cream Puffs, 113
  Banana Pudding, 58
  Banana Split Napoleon, 34
  Banana Walnut Roll-Up, 66
  Banana Walnut Tart, 47
  Bananas and Yogurt, 18
  Frozen Bananas, 19
  Individual Banana Soufflés, 18-19
  Lime and Banana Gelatin Dessert, 104
  Orange Banana Smoothie, 14
  Pear and Banana Gelatin Dessert, 103
  Strawberry-Banana Cubes, 102-103
  Strawberry-Banana Frozen Yogurt, 16-27
  Tropical Banana Pops, 22-23
Basic Meringue, 70-74
Basic Roll-Up Recipe, 64
Berry Good Napoleon, 38
Blintz Filling for Crêpes, 60-61
blueberries
  Blueberry Sour Cream Pie, 128-129
  Blueberry-Yogurt Pie, 84
  Double Blueberry Pie, 85
  July 4th Tart, 51
  Marinated Blueberries, 20
Butter-Almond Frappé, 12
butter and oil replacement, 59, 83, 126, 133,
  135, 138
Butterscotch Pie, 96
butterscotch pudding mix, 54, 96
  Double Meringue Butterscotch Pie, 80
C
Café-au-Lait Squares, 106
cantaloupe, 108
Carrot Cake with Cream Cheese Icing, 134-135

Chambord liqueur, 75
cherries
  Cherry Bread Pudding, 141
  Cherry Cheese Suzette, 133
  Cherry Glaze, 30, 31
  Cherry Strudel Filling, 40
  Pistachio Pineapple Tart, 44
  Tangerine Tart, 48
  Valentine Tarts, 72
cherry liqueur, 125
chocolate
  candy, 19, 54
  Chocolate Charlotte, 121
  Chocolate Chocolate Pie, 97
  Chocolate Dream Torte, 79
  Chocolate Frappé, 12
  Chocolate Glaze, 34, 35, 111
  Chocolate Mayonnaise Cake, 131
  Chocolate Mousse Pudding, 52, 111
  Chocolate Pear Tart, 46
  Chocolate Raspberry Tart, 46-47
  Chocolate Roll-Up, 65
  Chocolate Tart Filling, 44-45, 46, 121
  Frozen Chocolate Cream Puffs, 115
  Mocha Tart Filling, 32R, 67
  pudding mix, 52, 65, 79, 97
Cocoa Chiffon Pie, 99
coconut, 48, 90, 98
coconut extract, 108
coffee
  Coffee-and-Cream Pie, 98
  Mocha Frappé, 15
  Mocha Glaze, 33
  Mocha Mousse Pudding, 52-53
cottage cheese
  Blintz Filling for Crêpes, 60-61
  Blueberry-Yogurt Pie, 84
  Cherry Cheese Suzette, 133
  Orange Cottage Cheese Dessert, 107
  Tiramisu, 118-119
cream cheese
  Butterscotch Pie, 96
  Chocolate Chocolate Pie, 97
  Cocoa Chiffon Pie, 99
  Cream Cheese Icing, 134, 135
  Cream Cheese Pastries, 139
  Double Blueberry Pie, 85
  Hawaiian Alaska, 83
  Langues de Chat, 130-131
  Peach Cream Cheese Pie, 91
  Raspberry Ribbon Pie, 89
  Raspberry Shimmer Pie, 88
  Rich Lemon Shorties, 132
  Strawberry Cream Cheese Pie, 93

Strawberry Cream Cheese Tart, 43
Tangerine Cream Tarts, 93
Cream Puff Pastry, 110-116
Cream Puffs with Raspberry Sauce, 114
"Creamsicle" Gelatin, 109
Creamy Melon Gelatin
Crêpes Marcelles, 63
Cupcakes with a Cherry on Top, 138
Custard, Quick, 56
Custard Pie, Quick, 129
D
Deep Dish Pie Shell, 126, 127-130
Double Blueberry Pie, 85
Double Meringue Butterscotch Pie, 80
E
Easy Mixed Fruit-Gelatin Dessert, 106-107
Eggnog, Icy, 13
egg whites, 94, 140, 70
egg yolks, 69, 84, 86, 128
  Tiramisu, 118-119
equipment, 8
F
fillo dough. See phyllo dough
French Raspberry Pavlova, 76
Fresh Strawberry Roll-Up, 64-65
Fried Spiced Apples, 20
Frozen Bananas, 19
Frozen Chocolate Cream Puffs, 115
Frozen Pumpkin Pie, 95
Frozen Raspberry Cream Puffs, 116
Frozen Strawberry Cream Puffs, 116
Frozen Strawberry Mousse, 27
Frozen Watermelon Pops, 22
G
gelatin, unflavored, 17, 84, 86, 91, 96, 98,
  99, 106, 108
gelatin mixes, 8
ginger ale, 101
Ginger-Strawberry Cooler, 101
Gourmet Strawberries and Mint, 118
Grand Marnier liqueur, 122
H
Hawaiian Alaska, 83
Hawaiian Napoleon, 29
Hawaiian Pineapple Pie, 90-91
honeydew melon, 108
  Honeydew Sherbet, 24
hot chocolate
  Chocolate Frappé, 12
  Mocha Frappé, 15
  Quick Mocha Mousse, 53
Hot Fudge Napoleon, 36
I
Icy Eggnog, 13

Icy Peach Cream Puffs, 115
Individual Banana Soufflés, 18-19
Individual Strawberry Trifles, 122-123
J
Jamaican Trifle, 122
July 4th Tart, 51
K
Kaiser Schmarren, 62
Key Lime Pudding, 104-105
kiwifruit
  New Zealand Cream Puffs, 114
  Pavlova Wedges with Kiwis and Raspberry
  Sauce, 74-75
  Strawberry-Kiwi Tart, 49
L
Langues de Chat, 130-131
lemon
  gelatin mix, 24, 87, 105
  Lemon Chiffon Pie, 87
  Lemon Filling for Berry Good Napoleon,
  38, 39
  Lemon Ice Cream, 24
  Lemon Meringue Kisses, 77
  Lemon Meringue Torte, 78
  Lemon Pudding, 105
  Lemon Sauce, 124-125R
  Lemon Sponge Pudding, 56
  Lemony Angel Food, 123
  pudding mix, 78, 124
Light Chocolate Cream Puffs, 111
Light Mocha Cream Puffs, 111
Lime and Banana Gelatin Dessert, 104
Lime Chiffon Pie, 86-87
lime gelatin powder, 70-71, 86-87, 104
  Creamy Melon Gelatin Dessert, 108
  Key Lime Pudding, 104-105
  Lime Kisses, 70-71
M
Marinated Blueberries, 20
melons
  Creamy Melon Gelatin Dessert, 108
  Frozen Watermelon Pops, 22
  Honeydew Sherbet, 24-25
Meringue Chantilly, 80-81
meringues, 69-83
meringues, tips, 69
Microwave Vanilla Pudding, 57
Mixed Fruit Sherbet, 26
Mocha Cream Puffs, 112
Mocha Frappé, 15
Mocha Glaze, 33, 112
Mocha Mousse Pudding, 52-53
Mocha Napoleon, 32
Mocha Raspberry Roll-Up, 67

Mocha Tart Filling, 32, 67, 111, 112
N
Napoleon Fudge Topping, 37, 111, 112
Napoleons
  Banana Split Napoleon, 34
  Berry Good Napoleon, 38
  Hawaiian Napoleon, 29
  Hot Fudge Napoleon, 36
  Mocha Napoleon, 32
  Washington's Birthday Napoleon, 30-31
New Zealand Cream Puffs, 114
Not-Too-Sweet Chocolate Sauce, 55, 57
O
oranges
  "Creamsicle" Gelatin, 109
  Mixed Fruit Sherbet, 26
  Orange Banana Smoothie, 14
  Orange Cottage Cheese Dessert, 107
  Orange Frost, 25
  Oranges and Grapes, 21
  Orange Tart, 50
  Pineapple-Mint Drink, 11
  Yogurt Orange Whip, 17
orange gelatin mix
  Easy Mixed-Fruit Gelatin Dessert, 106-
    107
  Orange Cottage Cheese Dessert, 107
orange juice
  Apricot Filling for Strudel, 42
  Kaiser Schmarren, 62
  Orange-Glazed Coffee Cake, 136-137
  Orange Icing, 136, 137, 138
  Peach Cream Cheese Pie, 91
  Tart Orange Meringue Tarts, 71
Orange-Walnut Muffins, 140
P
Pavlova, Traditional, 74
Pavlova Wedges with Kiwis and Raspberry
  Sauce, 74-75
peaches
  Icy Peach Cream Puffs, 115
  Peach Charlotte, 120-121
  Peach Clafouti, 16
  Peach Cream Cheese Pie, 91
  Peach Crème Fraîche, 16-17
  Peach Melba Roll-Up, 66
  Peach Pavlova, 76-77
  Peach and Raspberry Tart, 48-49
pears
  Chocolate Pear Tart, 46
  Pear and Banana Gelatin Dessert, 103
pecans, 130
phyllo dough, 28-51
  strudels, 40-42

tarts, 42
tips, 28, 40, 42
pie crust, 84-86, 88-99, 127-130
Piña Colada Sherbet, 21
Piña Colada Squares, 108-109
pineapple
  Banana Split Napoleon, 34
  Crêpes Marcelles, 63
  Hawaiian Alaska, 83
  Hawaiian Napoleon, 29
  Hawaiian Pineapple Pie, 90-91
  Jamaican Trifle, 122
  Piña Colada Sherbet, 21
  Pineapple-Mint Drink, 11
  Pistachio Pineapple Roll-Up, 67
  Pistachio Pineapple Tart, 44
  Virgin Piña Colada, 13
pineapple juice
  Piña Colada Squares, 108-109
pistachio
  Pistachio Pineapple Roll-Up, 67
  Pistachio Pineapple Tart, 44
Prune Filling for Strudel, 41
pumpkin
  Butterscotch Pie, 96
  Frozen Pumpkin Pie, 95
  Pumpkin Ice Cream Pie, 94-95
  Thanksgiving Pumpkin Mousse, 54
Q
Quick Custard Pie, 129
Quick (and Foolproof) Mocha Mousse, 53
Quick (Microwave) Custard, 56-57
R
raspberries
  Berry Good Napoleon, 38
  French Raspberry Pavlova, 76
  Mocha Raspberry Roll-Up, 67
  Peach and Raspberry Tart, 48-49
  Raspberry Cream Gelatin, 100
  Raspberry Cream Pie, 90
  Raspberry Filling for Raspberry Cream
    Pie, 90, 116
  Raspberry Frappé, 15
  Raspberry Ribbon Pie, 89
  Raspberry Sauce, 74, 75, 114
  Raspberry Shimmer Pie, 88
raspberry jam
  Mocha Napoleon, 32
raspberry preserves
  Austrian Raspberry Cream Crêpes, 61
  Chocolate Charlotte, 121
  Chocolate Raspberry Tart, 46-47
  Raspberry Sauce, 75
Rich Lemon Shorties, 132

ricotta cheese
  Orange-Glazed Coffee Cake, 136-137
  Ricotta Cheese Pudding, 54-55
  Tiramisu, 118-119
Roll-Up (Cake) Basic Recipe, 64
S
Schaum Torte, 81
Snowball Cake, 117
  Sour Cream Pie, 130
Squash Pie, 128
strawberries
  Berry Good Napoleon, 38
  Fresh Strawberry Roll-Up, 64-65
  Frozen Strawberry Mousse, 27
  Gourmet Strawberries and Mint, 118
  Individual Strawberry Trifles, 122-123
  July 4th Tart, 51
  Mixed Fruit Sherbet, 26
  New Zealand Cream Puffs, 114
  Schaum Torte, 81
  Snowball Cake, 117
  Strawberries Chantilly, 125
  Strawberry-Banana Cubes, 102-103
  Strawberry-Banana Frozen Yogurt, 26-27
  Strawberry Bombe, 82
  Strawberry Charlotte, 120
  Strawberry Cream Cheese Pie, 93
  Strawberry Cream Cheese Tart, 43
  Strawberry Cream Puffs, 113
  Strawberry Ice Cream Pie, 92
  Strawberry Ice Cream Pie Filling, 92, 116
  Strawberry-Kiwi Glaze, 29, 30
  Strawberry-Kiwi Tart, 49
  Strawberry Layered Dessert, 102
  Strawberry Meringue Pie, 94
  Strawberry Smoothie, 14
  Strawberry Trifles, Individual, 122-122
  Strawberry Yogurt Dessert, 100-101

Traditional Pavlova, 74
strawberry-banana gelatin mix
  Banana Cream and Strawberry Pie, 92-93
  Pear and Banana Gelatin Dessert, 103
Sweet Crêpe Batter, 60-63
Sweet Potato Pie, 127
T
tangerine juice, 73
tangerines
  Tangerine Cream Tarts, 73
  Tangerine Tart, 48
Tart Orange Meringue Tarts, 71
Thanksgiving Pumpkin Mousse, 54
Tiramisu, 118-119
Tortoni, 23
Traditional Cream Puffs, 112
Traditional Pavlova, 74
Tropical Banana Pops, 22-23
V
Valentine Tarts, 72
Vanilla Pudding, Microwave, 57
Vanilla Shake, 11
Vanilla Tart Filling, 45, 47-51, 63, 66, 76,
  77, 112, 113, 114, 120
Virgin Piña Colada, 13
W
Walnut Roll-up Cookies, 99
Washington's Birthday Napoleon, 30-31
Watermelon Pops, Frozen, 22
white topping, 65, 71, 107
Y
yogurt
  Bananas and Yogurt, 18
  Gourmet Strawberries and Mint, 118
  Raspberry Frappé, 15
  Strawberry-Banana Frozen Yogurt, 26-27
  Strawberry Yogurt Dessert, 100
  Yogurt Orange Whip, 17